ESSENTIAL OILS FOR BEGINNERS

The Young Living Book Guide of Natural Remedies for Beginners

(Discover the Magic Power of Essential Oils)

Jeffrey McKenzie

Published by Tomas Edwards

© **Jeffrey McKenzie**

All Rights Reserved

Essential Oils for Beginners: The Young Living Book Guide of Natural Remedies for Beginners (Discover the Magic Power of Essential Oils)

ISBN 978-1-990268-98-4

All rights reserved. No part of this guide may be reproduced in any form without permission in writing from the publisher except in the case of brief quotations embodied in critical articles or reviews.

Legal & Disclaimer

The information contained in this book is not designed to replace or take the place of any form of medicine or professional medical advice. The information in this book has been provided for educational and entertainment purposes only.

The information contained in this book has been compiled from sources deemed reliable, and it is accurate to the best of the Author's knowledge; however, the Author cannot guarantee its accuracy and validity and cannot be held liable for any errors or omissions. Changes are periodically made to this book. You must consult your doctor or get professional medical advice before using any of the suggested remedies, techniques, or information in this book.

Upon using the information contained in this book, you agree to hold harmless the Author from and against any damages, costs, and expenses, including any legal fees potentially resulting from the application of any of the information provided by this guide. This disclaimer applies to any damages or injury caused by the use and application, whether directly or indirectly, of any advice or information presented, whether for breach of contract, tort, negligence, personal injury, criminal intent, or under any other cause of action.

You agree to accept all risks of using the information presented inside this book. You need to consult a professional medical practitioner in order to ensure you are both able and healthy enough to participate in this program.

Table of Contents

INTRODUCTION 1

CHAPTER 1: LAVENDER LINEN SPRAY 4

CHAPTER 2: HEALTHY ESSENTIAL OIL RECIPES FOR WEIGH LOSS 8

- DIY WEIGHT LOSS RECIPES 8
- WEIGHT LOSS SHOT 10
- SLIMMING BEVERAGE 11
- WEIGHT PROBLEMS 12

CHAPTER 3: ABUNDANT HEALTH RECIPES 15

- PMS BATH 15
- BUG BITES AND SUNBURNS 16
- IMMUNE BOOSTER 17
- STUFFY NOSE 17
- BLOOD PRESSURE REDUCER 18
- RELAXATION INDUCER 19
- ATHLETE'S FOOT 19
- PREMENSTRUAL CRAMPS 20
- REDUCE BINGE-EATING 20
- COLD AND FLU 21
- QUIT SMOKING 21
- CONSTIPATION 22
- STRESS RELIEF 23
- EAR INFECTION 24
- BRAIN BOOST 24

CHAPTER 4: BENEFITS OF AROMATHERAPY AND ITS APPLICATIONS 26

CHAPTER 5: ESSENTIAL OILS FOR BETTER IMMUNITY 31

CHAPTER 6: WHAT ARE ESSENTIAL OILS 37

CHAPTER 7: FACTORS TO CONSIDER WHEN BUYING ESSENTIAL OILS 42

CHAPTER 8: WHAT ARE ESSENTIAL OILS? 49

CHAPTER 9: WHAT ARE ESSENTIAL OILS? 52

CHAPTER 10: ESSENTIAL OILS AND THEIR BENEFITS 59

CHAPTER 11: ALL ABOUT ESSENTIAL OILS......................... 80

CHAPTER 12: HOW TO USE ESSENTIAL OILS..................... 89

CHAPTER 13: DIY NON-TOXIC CLEANING PRODUCTS....... 98

CHAPTER 14: WHAT ARE ESSENTIAL OILS? 107

CHAPTER 15: THE POWER OF SMELL 114

CHAPTER 16: THE MOST EFFECTIVE ESSENTIAL OILS FOR WEIGHT LOSS AND RECIPES... 123

GRAPEFRUIT ESSENTIAL OIL 124
LEMON ESSENTIAL OIL.. 127
ROOM SPRAY 129
FAT-BURNING TRIO FOR INTERNAL USE 132
CRISPY CINNAMON BAKED APPLE CHIPS RECIPE 134
TENSION TAMER BATH SALT RECIPE 140

EASY LAVENDER NECK RUB 146

CHAPTER 17: BENEFITS OF ESSENTIAL OILS 150

CHAPTER 18: ESSENTIAL OILS FOR INSECT BITE AND REPELLENT SPRAY 157

CHAPTER 19: TYPES OF ESSENTIAL OILS......................... 161

CHAPTER 20: THE POWER OF NATURE: DANGERS AND SAFETY 167

CHAPTER 21: ROSEMARY ESSENTIAL OIL 176

CONCLUSION.. 197

Introduction

We have recipes for cleaning your home, for helping out with minor ailments, to help boost immunity, to keep skin radiant, for baby, for mommy, for little sis and big brother and even for the family pet - this is a compendium packed with recipes that will help make you and your loved ones healthier, looking great and happier overall.

All you need to do is to go to the section that interests you and choose the recipe that you like the most, get the ingredients and cook up a cure in your own kitchen.

If you are a beginner when it comes to using essential oils, this book puts recipes devised by expert aroma-therapists over the years and step by step instructions at your fingertips. Think of it as a massive cheat sheet - you get to get all the benefits without needing to worry about trial and error or wasting time.

If, on the other hand, you already know something about how essential oils work and what properties they hold, you don't need to go over all of that again. This book is perfect for you - packed with recipes that you can try at your leisure without all the explanatory stuff that you have seen hundreds of times before.

Whether you are a beginner or an expert, this book will provide new recipes that you can try and have fun

The aim here is to provide you with recipes that you can use so we haven't added sections on safety protocols. As a result, I advise that you use the recipes as they are laid out in the book, making no substitutions unless you know a good deal about mixing essential oil blends and safety when using essential oils.

Essential oils are potent and, when used in the correct dilutions can be an extremely useful tool. When used in dilutions that are too high, however, problems can come about.

If you feel as though you would like to adjust the recipes, I advise that you keep the dilutions the same - double or triple a recipe if you like, but do keep the basics the same.

If you want to swap out one oil for another, I advise you to do some more research into properly blending oils - especially when it comes to oils used on your child or pets.

Chapter 1: Lavender Linen Spray

This can be a light splash that makes your clothing smell amazing and helps protect your health. After drying your clothes or sheets, spray or splash them with this Lavender Linen Spray for a wonderful and comforting aroma that will follow you all day. Since Lavender oil is gently, it is safe to use on your children's sheets before bed time. You could likewise utilize this as a relaxing body oil or fragrance (trade the refined water with light transporter oil like extracted coconut oil.)

What you'll need:

2 ounce dim glass splash bottle

1 teaspoon of witch hazel

15-20 drops of Lavender oil

Nearly 2 ounces of refined water

Instructions:

Put the Lavender in your glass bottle. Add the witch hazel. Fill the rest of the bottle with refined water. Put on the splash top and shake bottle vigorously. Sprinkle on crisply washed pieces of clothing or on your mattress and sheets shortly before sleeping.

Cheats Spray

This flavourful oil mix smells like Christmas. I love this Cheats splash crucial oil formula and like to share it with my family and friends. It's easy to use, and I have one in my home and one in my diaper pack for travel.

You can use it to:

Clean children's toys

Clean public restroom seats

Wipe down cutting boards

Wash leafy foods

Freshen gym bags

Disinfect plane armrests and serving plates

Spray inside the room to get rid of overwhelming smells

The uses of this spray are especially ceaseless. Also, it's super easy to make.

What you'll need:

2 oz. Darkish glass splash bottle

1 teaspoon common witch hazel

10-15 drops of youthful living Cheats oil

Almost 2 oz. of refined water

Instructions:

For your perfect splash bottle, add 10-15 drops of your Cheats oil. Then add 1 tsp of witch hazel. Top up the bottle with refined water. . That is it! That is one of my favorite DIY crucial oil formulas!

Glossy Hair Serum

Who doesn't want thick, striking and magnificent hair? Generally because of stress,baby blues or age, our hair can start to thin, break or lose its radiance. I truly enjoy utilizing this DIY crucial oil formula to improve how my hair looks and smells.

What you'll need:

2 ounce darkish glass dropper bottle

Close to 2 ounces of castor oil

10 drops of rosemary essential oil

5 drops of lavender crucial oil

5 drops of ylang premier oil

Instructions:

Pour 2 oz. of Castor Oil into your dropper bottle. Add the remaining oils. Put on dropper cover and shake bottle. Rub the mixture into your hair every morning. Leave it for up to 20 minutes then wash. It can be applied before bed, too! If you find the serum too oily, replace the castor oil with 2 oz. of refined water and 1 teaspoon of witch hazel.

Chapter 2: Healthy Essential Oil Recipes For Weigh Loss

Diy Weight Loss Recipes

There are countless essential oil recipes for weight loss. This chapter lists some of the most widely used recipes that, when accompanied with a healthy lifestyle, will enable you to reach your weight loss goals.

Keep in mind that essential oils are dense and highly concentrated. If you plan on applying essential oils topically, avoid doing so in their undiluted form. Dilute the essential oil first with a carrier oil of your choice to make the oil mild enough for topical application.

This blend takes four key essential oils and combines their powerful effects into one effective oil blend for shedding body fat. If your budget doesn't allow for a visit to an aromatherapist, this blend is a relatively inexpensive alternative—and incredibly easy to make, too.

Recipe:
5 drops of peppermint essential oil
10 drops of bergamot essential oil
10 drops of sandalwood essential oil
15 drops of grapefruit essential oil
A ceramic bowl
A clean spoon
A dark tinted glass vial
Carrier oil as needed

Directions:
Start by combining all of the essential oils in a clean bowl, and mix well.
Carefully pour the blend into a vial. Shake well.
Use ten drops of the blend for every bath, making sure to soak for at least 30 minutes while massaging the areas of your body where fat tends to accumulate.
For a quick massage, simply dilute 1-2 drops of the essential oil blend in an ounce of almond, jojoba, coconut, or extra virgin olive oil. Massage the mixture into your cellulite-prone areas, your forehead, the back of your neck, or your feet.

This special blend also works great in your diffuser. 6-8 drops should do the trick.

Weight Loss Shot

The last thing you need if you're trying to shed a few unwanted pounds is alcohol. However, this recipe allows you to take shots without harming your health. It includes absolutely zero alcohol— just the slimming and therapeutic benefits of three essential oils. This shot improves metabolism and digestion, significantly reduces stress and wards off midday and midnight cravings. It offers approximately one week of use, so feel free to double or triple the ingredients for prolonged usage.

Recipe:
5 drops of either grapefruit or lemon essential oil
5 drops of bergamot essential oil
5 drops of frankincense essential oil
A tinted glass vial with dropper

Directions:

Add all three essential oils in a vial and shake to combine.

Fill a shot glass with water or fresh orange juice. Add 1-2 drops of the oil blend. Bottoms up!

Repeat three times a day before each meal, or anytime stress or cravings raise their ugly heads.

Slimming Beverage

This recipe combines five weight-reducing essential oils for the ultimate weight loss drink. It works great as an appetite suppressant and is mild enough to drink throughout the day. In fact, it is recommended to drink this beverage as often as four times a day as essential oils are quickly absorbed and utilized by your body.

Supplying your body with a consistent flow of essential oils is important for ultimate efficacy. This beverage also promotes sleep: proper rest is a key tool for any weight loss plan.

Recipe:

20 drops of cinnamon essential oil (Make sure to use essential oil derived from cinnamon bark.)

40 drops of grapefruit essential oil

40 drops of lemon essential oil

40 drops of ginger essential oil

40 drops of peppermint essential oil

A 15ml tinted glass vial with dropper

Directions:

Put all of the essential oils into a vial and shake to combine well. Your vial should be nearly full once you've added all of the ingredients.

Before each meal, dilute two drops of the oil blend in a glass cup of cool mineral water, and drink.

Weight Problems

You are overweight.

Do you want to get rid of those unsightly bulges?

Cypress is effective against fat deposits and cellulite. It is also excellent for vascular drainage. Lemon grass is a tonic which stimulates and decongests veins. Juniper promotes active metabolism. Mint refreshes and stimulates circulation

Recipe:
After showering, massage with the following preparation:
100 ml of avocado oil
20 drops of essential oil of cypress
20 drops of essential oil of lemon grass
20 drops of essential oil of juniper
10 drops of essential oil of mint.

Directions:
Place a few drops of cypress in your ear overnight. This will promote weight loss. Above all, during your diet, choose foods which are light, rich in fiber and contain little fat and sugar. Cut your daily intake by half, keep moving, walk upstairs instead of taking the lift, skip around, and be active.

Take good care of yourself. You are an important person and nothing should trouble you.

Chapter 3: Abundant Health Recipes

There are several ways that essential oils can help with your health. They can alleviate illnesses like athlete's foot, acne, and can even help boost your immunity when you have a cold.

Your health is what keeps your body moving, gives you energy, and just keeps you alive. It is a very important part of your life, and if you're looking for a way to increase your health you're in the right place.

Here are few ways you can improve your health with the help of essential oils.

Pms Bath

Ingredients:
3 drops geranium oil
4 drops ylang ylang oil
4 drops Clary sage oil
1 teaspoon massage or olive oil
Instructions:

Fill the bath with warm water and add in all the ingredients. Stir the oils into the water before entering. Soak in the water for about 30 minutes, allowing the aromas from the oils to penetrate your nose.

Bug Bites And Sunburns

Ingredients:
4 oz. bottle
Nature's Fresh
Powdered vitamin C Ascorbates
4 drops lavender oil
1 to 2 drops Helichrysum oil
Instructions:
Fill the bottle most of the way with the Nature's Fresh. Add in all the ingredients and shake. Add to your bug bites and sunburns. The Helichrysum oil does not need to be added but it helps relieve pain and increases healing speed. This can be taken on camping and rafting trips to help your spots right away, so make sure your container is easy to take with you.

Immune Booster

Ingredients:
40 drops lavender oil
20 drops Tea Tree oil
10 drops Roman Chamomile oil
10 drops lemon oil
Carrier oil (such as almond or coconut), or massage oil

Instructions:
Mix all the ingredients into whatever air tight container you want. Apply close to the nose so you can inhale the scent. This recipe can also be used in a bath if you choose. You can also place in a diffuser to increase the immunity of everyone in a room. This is especially good for those with multiple kids who always get sick together, one right after the other.

Stuffy Nose

Ingredients:

6 drops Eucalyptus oil
3 drops lemon oil
3 drops Neroli oil
Instructions:
Mix all the oils into your choice container. Apply close to the nose until stuffy nose is gone. This recipe can also be used in the bath or a diffuser, just as long as you inhale the scent. If you choose to place in a container you can take it with you when you go and have relief on the go.

Blood Pressure Reducer

Ingredients:
10 drops lemon oil
10 drops sweet marjoram oil
10 drops ylang ylang oil
30 drops Clary sage oil
Instructions:
Mix all the ingredients together and apply on the skin. The best places are on the bottom of the feet or on the upper chest, near the neck. Apply daily or when you begin to have issues.

Relaxation Inducer

Ingredients:
50 drops mandarin oil
25 drops lavender oil
12 drops sweet marjoram oil
5 drops sandalwood oil
Instructions:
Mix all the oils together and apply near the nose. You can also apply on the bottom of the feet. This recipe can be used in a diffuser, and is not recommended for extended baths. You may fall asleep in the bath if used for an extended time.

Athlete's Foot

Ingredients:
5 drops massage oil
2 drops Tea Tree oil
1 drop lavender oil
Instructions:

Mix all the ingredients in your hand and massage onto feet and between toes. Wash hands after use. Apply to the feet at least twice a day. Use until you're Athlete's foot is completely gone.

Premenstrual Cramps

Ingredients:
10 drops ylang ylang oil
10 drops Clary sage oil
10 drops lavender oil
Instructions:
Fill your bathtub with warm water and add in all the oils. Mix the oils before entering. Soak at least once a day when symptoms are present. Try soaking for about 30 minutes to truly relieve the pain and allow the oils to soak into the skin.

Reduce Binge-Eating

Ingredients:
10 drops Clary sage oil

10 drops ylang ylang oil
Instructions:
These two oils will boost your self-confidence, making it so you don't want to binge-eat. You can apply this recipe to the bottom of your feet or bathe in it. It's best used when you have the cravings to eat when you don't need to.

Cold And Flu

Ingredients:
10 drops Eucalyptus oil
10 drops pine oil
Instructions:
Mix the oils together either in a daily bath or add to a diffuser. This recipe is best inhaled. Place some on your pillow at night where you can smell it as well to help clear up that cold. Use this recipe until your cold clears up and you feel you no longer need it.

Quit Smoking

Ingredients:
10 drops massage or carrier oil (sweet almond or coconut oil)
10 drops thyme oil
10 drops ylang ylang oil
10 drops pine oil

Instructions:
Add the carrier or massage oil to a container. Add in the other oils and stir gently. Rub near your nose and keep excess nearby so you can inhale often. This simulates the smell of smoking so instead of taking in dangerous chemicals you're inhaling something beneficial. This is a great substitute in places where smoking is not permitted. You can add this recipe to a diffuser as well.

Constipation

Ingredients:
15 drops rosemary oil
10 drops lemon oil
5 drops peppermint oil

2 tablespoons massage or vegetable oil
Instructions:
Mix the massage oil and the essential oils together. Rub this mixture on your lower abdomen in a counter-clockwise motion. Apply three times a day until constipation clears.

Aching Joints

Ingredients:
10 to 20 drops Eucalyptus oil
Instructions:
Fill your tub with warm water and add in the Eucalyptus oil. Stir before entering and soak for about thirty minutes.

Stress Relief

Ingredients:
30 drops bergamot oil
10 drops geranium oil
10 drops ylang ylang oil
Instructions:

Mix all the oils together and either add to a diffuser or rub onto the bottom of the feet.

Ear Infection

Ingredients:
1 teaspoon massage oil
3 drops Tea Tree oil
1 drop thyme oil
2 drops lavender oil
Instructions:
Mix together the oils and apply around the ear, down the neck, and across the cheekbone. This follows the path of the infection so it can help clear up the whole thing.

Brain Boost

Ingredients:
7 drops massage oil
5 drops rosemary oil
1 drop peppermint oil

Instructions:

Mix the oils in your hand. Apply around the face, taking care not to get it in your eyes. Also rub on your neck, and if there is any remaining oil left rub into both hands. This will help pep up your brain and give you a boost.

Chapter 4: Benefits Of Aromatherapy And Its Applications

Aromatherapy can be quite beneficial for your well-being from both inside and out. If it is carried out in the proper way, it can help deal with many ailments which might afflict your body.

The human body is nearly always dealing with some problem or the other whether it is physical or psychological. Finding a holistic way to deal with these is how aromatherapy can help you.

When it comes to beauty concerns, aromatherapy has garnered a lot of positive reviews. Using these natural essential oils is a very holistic way to improve appearance. Instead of using chemical products sold commercially, all you use are these pure ingredients from nature. It works internally and thus has better results externally. Instead of opting for over rated products or expensive procedures, just implement some aromatherapy into your life. There are a lot of oils which will benefit you in various ways and give you a healthier appearance than ever before.

Aromatherapy does not just deal with your problems in a short terms and external way. The effects are long term and deep rooted hence more effective.

Listed below are some of the benefits that aromatherapy can have:

- Lifts mood while fighting depression and generates a feeling of well-being
- Helps to boost the immune system
- Can help to fight with bacterial or viral infections
- Improves sexual capacity and fertility
- Improves the appetite
- Relaxes the mind and soothes away anxiety and stress
- Helps to deal with sleeping problems and promotes a restful sleep
- Helps to relieve pain in the muscles and joints
- Helps to get blood pressure levels balanced
- It is good for hair growth and solving problems like dandruff or hair loss.

- Helps to improve the skin's appearance and texture. The oils can tone the skin and also treat problems like acne or eczema.
- There are no harmful chemicals and additives involved like in other methods. It is a pure and natural way of healing.
- It has long term benefits and works from inside unlike other methods.

Aromatherapy can be practicedin different ways. The essential oils can be used in a way for topical application or else through its olfactory stimulation. The oils work well for the body in terms of appearance as well as general well-being. It doesn't take much time to input some of these therapeutic practices into your daily life while the benefits are worth it.

Unlike commercial products, essential oils work extensively on the body and have long term benefits. They are also not just oriented towards one specific problem area and can benefit you in a variety of ways.

Aromatherapy has been practiced in different cultures in different ways to effectively solve many problems. They can solve skin problems like acne as well as improve internal health issues like indigestion or asthma. The symptoms of many diseases have shown to be reduced with the help of aromatherapy.

Find out what type your skin is and if any oils would have adverse effects on you. Patch tests or medical consultations can help you with this issue. Then accordingly utilize the oils with the various modes of application.

Modes of application of aromatherapy:

- Massage- This is a common way of applying the essential oils topically on the body. They are usually mixed with carrier oils and then used. The mixture is then rubbed into the body and soaked in. This is both a relaxing and effective way of utilizing the oils.

- Inhalation- Inhaling the essential oils is another common way of using them. Sometimes a few drops of the oil are just dropped into a cloth and held under the nose to breathe in the scent. Otherwise a few drops of the appropriate oil are dropped into a bowl of hot water. The steam is then inhaled from this.

- Bathing- The essential oils can also be used while bathing. A little oil can be poured into the bath and while you soak in it, the body soaks in the oils. Even vapors are produced from the heat and this is inhaled in. It is a relaxing and rejuvenating practice at the end of the day.
- Diffusion- Diffusers are available for this purpose. They help to diffuse the oils into the surroundings and this helps especially to deal with stress and respiratory problems.

Chapter 5: Essential Oils For Better Immunity

Essential oils are a plant's own safeguard against ailment; it does likewise for us when we apply it uniquely or in blend. Utilizing key oils that cooperate with other people of reciprocal nature is the heart of clinical fragrance based treatment, and this objective of collaboration can yield significant results in regards to the insusceptible framework. At the point when connected undiluted to the soles of the feet (the delicate, uncalloused part between the bundle of the foot and the heel), the antiviral-like properties of certain vital oils achieve the circulatory system inside 20 minutes and the most profound cell level inside a day.

Vital oils can help with the avoidance of getting the feared infections that bring about colds in a few distinctive ways. Utilizing fundamental oils, for example, Cinnamon, Clove, Eucalyptus, Lavender, Lemon, Sweet Orange and Thyme all discourage the development of infections and make them an astounding choice to use amid the months when most are inside because of cooler climate and windows are kept closed, restricting the measure of natural air flow. Vital oils are extremely flexible and can be diffused through a few intends to rinse and clean the air, and additionally perhaps add to raising your state of mind!

Wellbeing professionals prescribe that you keep five key oils close by to avoid or diminish the seriousness of a cool, hack, infection, fever or influenza. Oils such as lemon, peppermint and oregano are beneficial. An absolute must to have during flu season is a respiratory mix. This is mainly a blend of essential oils which include spruce, pine, myrtle, peppermint, marjoram oils and lavender along with three assortments of eucalyptus oil.

Breathing the oil into your sinuses and lungs can forestall or lighten the bodily fluid development from a frosty or a hack. Chilly air diffusers likewise secure the oil quality, not at all like warmth, which can harm the oil and make it less powerful.

You likewise can heat up any size pot of water, include four or five drops of oil to the bubbled water, cover your head with a towel and, while holding your head over the fluid, let the steam enter your sinuses and lungs. The oils, conveyed by the steam water atoms, will begin to discharge and kill the pathogens that have taken living arrangement in these territories.

For influenza you can apply the oil in strokes to the back, right beside the spine. The skin retains the oil rapidly as key oils normally enter the cell divider and work inside the cell. After experiencing speedier recovery, I do recommend putting a drop or two of oil on a warm washcloth and after that setting the washcloth on your mid-section to simplicity mid-section colds. I would also recommend rubbing some oil straightforwardly on your mid-section or back to battle a cool or an infection.

Invulnerable boosting vital oils can be your best partner consistently, yet in the event that you need to prepare for influenza season this winter, it is best to protective layer your body now while summer is still here. Here is a rundown of key oils you will need close by and why.

Clove Bud is probably one of the most capable and dependable crucial oils in clinical fragrance based treatment, clove battles infectious maladies and is an astounding oil to use for any bacterial, viral, or parasitic contamination. Likewise profoundly prescribed for Lyme sickness.

Eucalyptus citriodora is a standout amongst the most important. It has powerful against viral, hostile to bacterial, and against parasitic properties and is exceedingly successful for bacterial and viral contaminations of the respiratory framework

Eucalyptus globulus is a rich in menthol oil. Eucalyptus facilitates the torment of muscles and a joint connected with flu and fortifies the insusceptible framework to battle infections and microscopic organisms. It likewise battles irresistible fevers. Eucalyptus separates mid-section clog when weakened and connected to the mid-section and throat in non-asthmatics.

Lavender may seem to be a lightweight oil, however it is a vital oil to have close by at home keeping in mind voyaging. The most effective method to utilize: 4 drops undiluted on every sole of the foot. Works surprisingly better when layered with natural lemon vital oil.

Pine needle is great companion for viral exhaustion and hurting, winter muscles when a frosty or influenza is dragging you down.

Organic lemon vital oil is a standout amongst the strongest oils and the first to go to when one's safety is traded off. Natural lemon animates white platelet creation and helps safety against genuine diseases including pneumonia and staph.

Tea Tree Oil is capable and solid oil for the safe framework that is best when joined with natural lemon, white thyme, clove, or lavender vital oil to battle diseases and this season's cold virus.

There are many crucial oils, and even that apparently similar offer one of a kind advantage. With a little practice and considerably more learning, clinical fragrance based treatment can be utilized to drastically support invulnerability and prepare for winter sicknesses and much more prominent dangers. It is likewise flawless, fragrant approach to better wellbeing. Whenever you have a feeling that you're becoming ill, maybe consider one of these fundamental oils formulas for a characteristic street to recuperation.

Chapter 6: What Are Essential Oils

Essential oils are plant extracts which have been created by steam distillation of plant material from a single botanical source. The essential oil is separated from the condensed steam, and nothing is added or taken away.

These plants contain therapeutic properties known to help with some health ailments. Such essential oils are used in clinical aromatherapy practice to help with physical problems (pain, arthritis, nausea, etc.), emotional problems (depression, anxiety, stress, etc.), skin care, weight loss and much more.

Both organic and non-organic essential oils have the same therapeutic properties because both are extracted from plants.

What is Aromatherapy

Aromatherapy is a therapy that uses essential oils and water-based colloids obtained from plant materials to promote physical, emotional and spiritual health and balance. According to the Canadian Federation of Aromatherapist, aromatherapy is the art and science of using essential oils for improving and maintaining health and beauty.

The actual word is "Aroatherapie," which was created in 1928 by Rene Murice Gattefosse, a French chemist while he was conducting an experiment. His hands were severely burned in a lab explosion, and he found that Lavender healed them.

How Essential Oils Work

According to Deepak Chopra, a Medical Doctor and leading international spiritual Guru, he explains that when you inhale a scent, the aroma travels directly to the hypothalamus. The hypothalamus is an organ in the brain responsible for regulating growth, sleep, emotional responses and more.

This aroma flows through the body's limbic system and into an area of the hippocampus; that is the part of the brain that's responsible for memory. This process is called neuro-associative conditioning, which is the body's ability to link a healing response to a particular smell.

The sense of smell connects you directly with your emotions, instincts, and memories. Studies performed by NYU LangoneMedical Center concluded that when specific aromas were inhaled through the nose, the symptoms of headaches, menstrual pain and respiratory infection subsided.

Another study performed by the University of Maryland Medical Center concluded that inhaling lavender, rose and frankincense alleviated anxiety, stress, and depression. Also, the use of peppermint subsided nausea and chamomile subsided the pain.

Essential oils follow three main pathways to gain entry to the body: inhalation, ingestion, and absorption through the skin.

Inhalation

Inhalation is the access via the nasal passages; it is usually the quickest efficient route in the treatment of emotional problems such as stress and depression.

This is because the nose has direct contact with the brain, which is responsible for triggering the effects of essential oils. Methods of inhalation include:

The use of tissues that contain 5 to 6 drops of essential oil placed inside the shirt, blouse or nightwear.

Hands. This is an excellent method, but should be confined to emergencies only and isn't suitable for children. Put 1 drop in your palm, rub both hands and place the hands over your nose avoiding the eyes, then take a deep nasal breath.

Bath. Putting essential oils into the tub is effective because not only do they come into gentle contact with the skin, but also they are inhaled at the same time. This is a double benefit.

Spray bottle. A quick way of freshening the air, it can be used in the house, car or by spraying yourself.

Diffusers and Vaporizers: The main difference between diffusers and vaporizers is that diffusers push all the essential oil molecules out at the same time, while vaporizers push the lightest essential oil molecules out first.

Steam Inhalation:You can fill a bowl with warm water and add a few drops, cover your head with a towel and inhale the aroma for around five minutes.

Candles: A true aromatherapy candle is made with pure essential oils and is made from beeswax or soy.

Ingestion

When essential oils are taken by mouth, knowledge of the ingredients of the essential oils is of paramount importance. This means it is essential to know the strength of concentration, the nature of any diluents used and the length of time for which it is to be taken. Most aroma therapists are cautious about using ingestion, because of the greater danger of an excessive dose reaching the liver than if done by external application.

Chapter 7: Factors To Consider When Buying Essential Oils

Using essential oils is actually one of the best things that you can do to improve your general health and also of those around you. They have an all round advantage from maintaining your health and your home and they are therefore the most useful products you can purchase. In order to make your experience with essential pleasant you should always focus on quality, healing properties and fragrance.

When purchasing essential oils there are certain things you should put in mind like what you want to use the essential oil for, the grade of oil you need and much more. If you plan to introduce the use of certain essential oils for your family, children and animals it is advised that you go for 100% pure therapeutic grade oils. There are a number of places that you can buy essential oils and there are also a range of plant types and essentials oil brands that one can choose from.

When you are choosing an essential oil it all depends on what you are looking to cure or prevent, how effective you would like them to be and lastly at what cost you plan to achieve your goals. The cost of essential oils varies greatly as some products provide much better quality over others. The factors which influence the cost of essential oils include; where the plant is sourced, how rare the plant is and also quality control measures taken by the distiller.

Poor quality essential oils or adulterated oils are not considered as therapeutic. This is because they can cause harmful side effects or provide minimal therapeutic benefit. Pure essential oils are those that contain only the concentrated aromatic compounds from the plant without any adulteration. The additives and adulterations that are added to essential oils to lower production costs can include some chemical dilutants, some synthetic oils, a mixture of cheap oil and expensive ones, alcohol etc.

Whether you are a professional aromatherapist or a first timer in using essential oils quality should always be a point of focus. There are some factors that affect the quality of essential oils and they are as highlighted below:-

The method of production.

Harvesting and cultivation methods.

The part of plant that was used.

The origin of the essential oil.

The climate under which the plant was grown and the time it was harvested.

How the oil is stored and for how long.

There are some factors that one should consider when buying essential oils:-

Proper packaging and also the labeling standards.

How experienced the company founders are.

When buying essential oils always ensure you are keen on words like "fragrance oil", words such as "nature identical oil" or even "perfumes oil" as these words indicates that what you see is actually not pure, or it is not single essential oil.

How the plants are grown, buying essential oils provided by local sustainable growers is better than buying organic because of highly quality due to personal care given by local growers.

You should put into consideration the distillation process of the oil because the best processes are the ones which alter the essential oils the least retaining the most therapeutic value.

One can also consider the price factor because for quality you have to pay a little work.

There is also the idea of the reputation of the company you buy your products, ensure that it has a good reputation in terms of their services, quality and also prices of their essential oils.

Therapeutic properties should also be considered and one should therefore be familiar with the healing properties of the given oil.

You should also consider the fragrance of the essential oil because no matter how useful the properties are. If you can't stand the fragrance you will rarely use it.

Application methods for essential oils

Pure essential oils have a wide range of therapeutic benefits and it is important to know that the method applied affects the outcome. What you need to put in mind is that almost no essential oil should be applied undiluted to the skin. Essential oils are usually applied in three ways i.e. aromatically, topically and internally.

In using essential oils there are certain symbols you should watch out for:-

Green symbol: shows that it is safe to use without dilution as directed.

Orange symbol: it requires moderate dilution for safety.

Red symbol: indicates the need for heavy dilution and with precaution taken.

Aromatically application

The aromatic application of essential oils is said to be the most popular. Aromatic applications entail more than just the idea of a good smell. We experience the positive properties of essential oils as they can be absorbed into our blood stream through inhalation. The essential oils are processed by the olfactory and the limbic system which is the same system that is responsible for our thinking, feelings and even memories helping one to feel calm and relaxed.

The aroma one inhales is of the same components as its oil. One can inhale essential oils by the use of certain specific devices and also through different techniques e.g. diffuser, dry evaporation, steam and spray.

Topically

Using essential oils topically is simple but can also be delicate. A number of essential oils can be used topically. However there is variation in usage because some have precautions for dilution or frequency. It is also very essential for you to know your skin type because if you have sensitive skin you are required to always dilute the oil. When you dilute it the effectiveness of the essential oil is not reduced and it actually helps to increase absorption rate by preventing evaporation and also decreases the risk of a skin reaction.

Internally

It is very important to note that only a few essential oils can be used internally and also not all people use them internally because it may have some side effects on them. There are some certain essential oils that are generally recognized as safe for internal use they still come with precautions. The things you should keep in mind when using essential oils internally are as highlighted below:-

Less is more.

Increase frequency before the drops.

Limit your daily drops.

Always dilute.

Some people should avoid applying it internally.

Chapter 8: What Are Essential Oils?

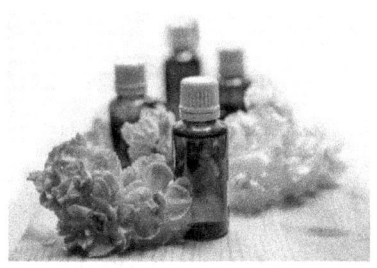

Essential oils are the essence of the herb, flower, or fruit rind. It is the most potent way to use herbals and other plant materials. They are made by either distilling the plant matter or pressing it. Essential oils are the mainstay ingredient in Aromatherapy blends and preparations.
What is Aromatherapy?
Aromatherapy is the practice of using aromas to improve, mood and health. It is also the practice of blending essential oils in different preparations to soothe aches, pains, and illness.

It works on the olfactory nerves and the limbic system of the brain. To make it simple, when you inhale an essential oil, your nose sends signals to the part of your brain that reacts emotionally.

This reaction can activate other systems in your body, like your immune system, to speed healing or it can send signals to your nerves to calm down, either relaxing you or helping relive nerve pain.

There are several applications of Aromatherapy, and all of them are all natural.

How much do essential oils cost?

This depends on the amount of plant material needed to make the oil and where the oil is made. For example, it takes a ton of rose petals to make half an ounce of rose essential oil. For this reason, it is one of the most expensive essential oils on the market. On the other hand, since peppermint is easy to come by, is more prevalent on the market and thus very affordable.

Are there any side effects?

If you are allergic to any of the plants, you are going to have a more severe allergic reaction to the essential oil. Also, be leery of any plants related to the ones you are allergic. Other than that, there really aren't any side effects to worry about.

Chapter 9: What Are Essential Oils?

Essential oils are obtained by a process of distillation by which the essence, life force, or 'spirit' of the plant is extracted by means of water or steam distillation, after which, the oil then is separated from the water. This oil is a concentrated pure form of the essence of the plant. For an essential oil to be characterized as a 'true' essential oil, it must have gone through this distillation process, and not merely blended with water and separated. There are a handful of 'essential' oils made from this second method, including bitter almond and spearmint, among others, yet they are not as powerful, concentrated, or considered to be of the same caliber as a true essential oil.

Essential oils contain all of the aroma compounds of the plant from which they have been distilled. This makes many of them very pleasant to smell as well as useful as vapors to be inhaled, since most essential oils are medicinal in nature, or at least health-inducing in some way. Most aroma-therapists agree that the term essential is a shortened version of quintessential, making the essential oil an example of the very plant it was derived from. Since essential oils are highly concentrated, generally only a few drops are needed. Some essential oils are so concentrated that in order to use them with the body they must be diluted by mixing them with a carrier oil.

What Can They Do For You?

Essential oils have numerous benefits to the human body. Used almost exclusively in aromatherapy, essential oils are added elements in alternative medicine because of the healing effects of their use. While some essential oils are claimed to have a relaxing effect on the body, others are thought to contribute to an uplifting or quickening of the mind and spirit.

While many essential oils have practical uses around the home, such as repelling insects, disinfecting countertops, and a host of other wonderful uses, for the purposes of our material, we will concentrate on the therapeutic properties of their fragrance.

There are so many different health benefits from using essential oils that we could barely scratch the surface of their practicality in one book, but we will look at some of the most popular types in our next chapter.

How Are Essential Oils Made?

There are three common methods of producing essential oils, the most common method that is employed today is known as distilling. A second method that is used produces a product that is considered less pure than distilling, and is called extraction, but produces a lesser quality of oil, as does the third method, known as expression. Since distilling produces the highest quality of essential oil, we will discuss the methods by which this type of essential oil is made.

Steam distillation is used to make many of the most common essential oils, including lavender, peppermint, tree, and eucalyptus, to name just a few. The raw material of the desired plant is placed in the distillation apparatus and set over boiling water. As the water is heated and boiled, the steam permeates the plant material, passes through it, and allows the volatile compounds in the plant to vaporize, after which, the vapors travel through the coil and condense back into liquid.

Almost all essential oils can be distilled in one single process such as this, however, a slight few require fractional distillation, which breaks up the process into several steps.

The Cost of Essential Oils

Essential oils range in cost from very reasonable to quite expensive, depending on the availability of the plant material and the demand for the oil on the market. Many of the more common essential oils can be purchased for a dollar for a third of an ounce bottle, as is the case for peppermint oil, while others, including the rare Champaca Absolute, can sell for over $2,000 per ounce. When purchasing essential oils, always be sure of the source and of the purity of the product, especially when investing in some of the more expensive oils. An unscrupulous marketer could cut an essential oil with a lesser quality oil without your knowledge, increasing their profit margin greatly, but giving you far less for your money. Buy from reputable companies that have a long history of satisfied customers.

Safety of Using Essential Oils

Essential oils are prized gifts from nature and must be handled with extreme caution, as their powerful nature is often greater than anticipated. Misuse of essential oils can cause harm to the skin, eyes, and body. Some 'hot' oils can cause a burning sensation to the skin, and should be tested on a small patch of skin before applying in a larger dose. These hot oils, such as cinnamon, are often mixed with a carrier oil that dilutes their essence to prevent skin burn.

Essential oils that cause redness of the skin or a rash should be discontinued immediately, diluted with a carrier oil, and carefully tested again in a different part of the body, once the initial reaction to the oil has subsided. If a reaction is noted as the result of a hot oil or other essential oil, use a carrier oil to wash away the essential oil and gently pat dry with a clean towel.

Essential oils should never be applied to the sensitive areas of the body including the eyes, ears, nostrils, genitals, or the mucous membranes. If you choose to ignore these guidelines and use essential oil in or near these particular parts of the body, dilute the essential oil with the ratio of one drop of essential oil to 10 - 20 drops of carrier oil.

With essential oil, consumers are often under the impression that since a small dose of oil brings good results, a large amount will bring better results. This is not the case with essential oils, which are potent and have the ability to heal, and to harm if carelessly used. The body seems to have a threshold that once crossed, proves to contribute to reactive problematic effects. In the case of essential oil, less is quite often more.

For use with children, always dilute the properties of the essential oil before applying or using, and always consult a specialist in essential oils before experimenting with the health of your child. Some of the more common oils, such as peppermint are considered quite safe in moderation. Using oils that you are not familiar with should warrant some special study on your part to keep your child safe.

Anytime you are using an essential oil for the first time for medicinal purposes, it is wise to study about the particular oil in question, consulting a professional or other experts to gain knowledge of what adverse effects may be associated with its use. When used carefully and properly, essential oils can be used in the home with many benefits.

Chapter 10: Essential Oils And Their Benefits

Essential oils offer a lot of benefits. They are commonly used for fragrance, incense, and as massage oil and mood lifter. Each essential oil offers various benefits and properties that can be used for different purposes.

These oils commonly blend with one another, resulting to a vast combination for various applications. They are combined either by their benefits or by their aroma. Take note that these are very potent oils and can cause irritation if you have sensitive skin or if you are allergic to fragrances. Do a skin patch test before using any essential oil to prevent any issues.

Allspice

This oil is extracted from Pimenta dioica of the Myrtaceae family and is also known as Jamica Pepper, Pimenta or Pimento Oil. It is an evergreen tree that can be found in South America and West Indies.

It has a warm feel with a spicy, sweet aroma. It tastes like a bit of clove combined with cinnamon, juniper berries and pepper. It is used to relieve pain, induce numbness, relax the body, stimulate body functions and add color to your skin. It is an analgesic, antiseptic, anesthetic, stimulant, and tonic, relaxant, carminative and rubefacient.

It blends well with geranium, ginger, orange, lavender, patchouli, clove, cassia, ylang ylang and cinnamon.

Angelica

Angelica has a sweet smell with a hint of spiciness. It is extracted from Angelica archangelica which is native in Eastern Europe. It usually blooms on the 8th of May which is St. Michael's Day, an archangel. Due to this, it is often planted in monasteries and is called Angel Grass, giving it its name, Angelica.

This oil helps boost the lymphatic system and detoxifies the body. It is also an effective treatment for respiratory issues and problems related to the stomach including dyspepsia, flatulence, indigestion, discomfort and nausea. It is also helpful for treating psoriasis, skin irritations, dull skin, gout, arthritis, rheumatism, bronchitis, water retention, cough, anorexia, anemia, fatigue, migraine, stress and nervous tension.

Although it blends with all essential oils aromatically, it does blend best with patchouli, mandarin, lemon, lavender, grapefruit, geranium, chamomile and basil. It is often used in burners and vaporizers, massage oil and bath water, or blended with creams and lotions.

Aniseed

This oil is warm and spicy and is extracted from the fruits and seeds of Pimpinella anisum which is an herb that originated in the Middle East. It is also known as sweet cumin but it must not be confused with star anise, although they have the same liqourice-like smell.

This oil is helpful for the digestive system, respiratory tract and circulatory system. It helps ease hangover, catarrh, flatulence, menstrual cramps, whooping cough, colic, bronchitis, muscle pains and rheumatism.

Use this oil with caution. Using it in large doses can cause cerebral congestion. Pregnant women should avoid using this oil.

It blends well with Cedarwood, cardamom, caraway, coriander, dill, mandarin, fennel, rosewood and petitgrain.

Basil

It has a very light yellowish to greenish color and has a sweet, peppery, green smell. It is often used in aromatherapy to clear the mind, steady the nerves, ease congested sinuses, cool down fever and treat menstrual issues.

It is used to treat bronchitis and asthma, as well as constipation, vomiting, nausea and hiccups. It generally refreshes the skin and is used for insect bites and acne.

It blends well with black pepper, bergamot, Cedarwood, ginger, fennel, geranium, grapefruit, lavender, marjoram, lemon, verbena and neroli.

Benzoin

It is resinous oil extracted from the Styrax Benzoin tree from Sumatra, Java and Thailand. It is also referred to as gum benzoin, Benjamin, luban jawi or styrax benzoin.

It has a golden-brown color with a warm, sweet vanilla-like aroma. It is calming oil that uplifts the spirit and the mind. It offers comfort to the sad and lonely. It also relieves cracked skin and improves its elasticity and heals sores, wounds irritation and itching. It is also used to treat acne, eczema, psoriasis, scar, digestive issues, circulation problems and respiratory tract problems.

It blends well with bergamot, frankincense, coriander, lavender, juniper, myrrh, lemon, petitgrain, orange, sandalwood and rose.

Bergamot

This fresh, citrus, fruity-sweet, spicy-floral oil is extracted from Citrus aurantium var. bergamia, also known as bergamot orange. It provides a relaxed, happy feeling, making it a favorite among aromatherapists.

It relieves stress, tension, depression, anorexia, hysteria and fear. It also helps treat psoriasis, eczema, oily skin, acne, chicken pox, wound and cold sores.

It blends well with black pepper, cypress, clary sage, frankincense, jasmine, geranium, nutmeg, mandarin, orange, sandalwood, rosemary, ylang-ylang and vetiver.

Black Pepper

This sharp, spicy smelling oil is extracted from Piper nigerum from the Piperaceae family. It warms the body and mind and stimulates circulation. It also promotes better digestion and stimulates the kidneys and colon. It also stimulates appetite and relieves sore muscles, pain and fever.

It blends well with bergamot, clove, clary sage, coriander, frankincense, fennel, ginger, geranium, grapefruit, lemon, lime, lavender, juniper, mandarin, sandalwood, sage and ylang-ylang.

Cajuput

It is extracted from Melaleuca cajuputi, an evergreen tree, also known as weeping tea tree, white wood or weeping paperback. It balances the mind, clears thoughts and dispels sluggishness. It has a sweet penetrating smell and is commonly used in perfumes and cosmetics.

It cools down the body by promoting perspiration and helps relieve bronchitis, laryngitis and colds. It also helps cure sore throat, sinusitis and asthma. It is also beneficial for the digestive system, rheumatism, arthritis and muscular pains. Its antiseptic properties help combat infections and skin conditions such as psoriasis and acne. It also relieves insect bites from lice and fleas and wards them off as well.

It blends well with bergamot, angelica, geranium, cloves, thyme and lavender.

Chamomile/Roman Camomile

It is extracted from Anthemis nobelis that belongs to the family species Asteraceae. It is also known as garden chamomile, sweet chamomile or English chamomile.

This oil is watery with a clear blue color and smells like sweet apple. It has a great calming effect, making it effective for children who are teething, irritable and impatient. It also relieves PMS, gall bladder issues, abdominal pain, allergies, throat infections, asthma and hay fever. It also helps relieve urinary stones and any type of inflammation.

It blends well with clary sage, bergamot, geranium, lavender, tea tree, jasmine, rose, grapefruit, ylang-ylang and lemon.

Camphor

This oil is extracted from the Camphor tree. Be cautious in choosing your camphor essential oil. Use only the white camphor that has a fresh, clear aroma. Do not use the yellow one as it contains safrole that is carcinogenic and toxic.

This oil balances your mood. It also sedates the nerves and uplifts apathy. It helps relieve inflammation, feeling cold, cough and bronchitis. It also effectively repels insects such as moths and flies. It also helps in reducing muscular pains, sprains, rheumatism and arthritis.

It blends well with cajuput, lavender, chamomile, basil and Melissa.

Cedarwood

This balsamic oil is extracted from Juniperus virginiana, also known as

Bedford Cedarwood Lebanon cedar. It is viscous with light yellow to pale orange color and a woody, pencil-like smell with a hint of sandalwood.

It is especially beneficial for the skin due to its sedating effect. It can cure acne, oily skin and itching. It is also effective for dandruff, chest infections and urinary infections. It also calms and soothes the mind, helping greatly in conditions associated with nervous tension and anxiety.

It blends well with bergamot, benzoin, cypress, cinnamon, jasmine, frankincense, juniper, lavender, neroli, lemon, rosemary and rose.

Cinnamon

It is extracted from Cinnamomum zeylanicum also known as true cinnamon, Ceylon or Seychelles. It has a musky, spicy warm smell that helps calm depression, relieve feeling of weakness and fights exhaustion.

In ancient Egypt, it is used as a foot massage, treatment for excessive bile and as temple incense. It is also used as sedative during birth and as a key ingredient for love potions and mulled wines.

This oil must be avoided during pregnancy due to its emmenagogue action. Only the oil from the leaf can be used for aromatherapy. The oil extracted from cinnamon bark can cause irritations, contains dermal toxins and a sensitizer.

It is used for clearing warts, calming the respiratory tract and the nervous system, and eases influenza and colds.

It blends well with cloves, coriander, benzoin, ginger, cardamom, frankincense, cloves, grapefruit, rosemary, lavender and thyme.

Citronella

This oil is extracted from a perennial, hardy grass native to Java and Sri Lanka. It is a known insect repellant and is also greatly used for clearing the mind, cleaning a sickroom, softening the skin, combats oily skin and relieves sweaty feet.

It has a citrusy, lemony smell with a hint of sweetness. It is popularly used for candles, perfumes, lotions, deodorants and soaps. It is also great for colds, infections and flu.

It blends well with geranium, bergamot, orange, lemon, pine and lavender.

Clary Sage

This oil is extracted from the leaves and flowering tops of the biennial herb. It is also known as clary wort, muscatel sage and see bright. It smells nutty and sweet with an herbaceous undertone.

It calms the nervous system, making it effective for treating depression, tension, insomnia and stress. It is also used as a relaxant during birth. It helps ease muscle pains, kidney diseases and digestive disorders. It also cools skin inflammation such as ulcers, boils and acne. It balances sebum production of the skin which removes grease and clears the complexion of your skin.

It blends well with lavender, juniper, pine, sandalwood, geranium, frankincense, jasmine and citrus oils.

Dill

This oil is extracted from the seeds or the entire plant. It is a biennial herb that is native from South West Asia. It has a very light yellow color and a grassy, nature-like smell.

It helps ease the feeling of being too overwhelmed and calms the mind. It is effective for digestive issues and also for hiccups. It also helps reduce excess sweating due to tension and nervousness. Breastfeeding moms can benefit from this oil as it helps increase breast milk production.

It blends well with citrus fruits as well as nutmeg and caraway and bergamot.

Eucalyptus

This oil is extracted from the Australian blue gum tree also known as Tasmanian blue gum. It has a distinctive, fresh, clear aroma that helps clear the mind and support better focus and concentration.

It is very helpful for migraines, fever, headaches, respiratory ailments, muscle pains and skin ailments such as skin ulcers, congested skin and wounds.

It blends well with thyme, benzoin, lemongrass, pine and lavender.

Fennel

This oil is extracted from the seeds of the perennial herb known as Sweet Fennel, Roman Fennel or Fenkle. Egyptians and Romans use fennel to strengthen their eyesight, as a cure for snakebite and remove fleas from dogs. It is also believed to ward off bad spirits, enhance strength and courage, and convey longevity.

It has an herby aroma with a hint of spiciness that resembles aniseed. When taken in large doses, it can have a narcotic effect and must be avoided in cases of epilepsy and pregnancy.

This essential oil is used for weight loss as it promotes the feeling of fullness and its diuretic effect helps the body get rid of toxins. In aromatherapy, it is used to boost one's courage and strength to face life's adversity. It also has estrogenic properties which help minimize wrinkles and clear the skin, balance oily skin, and speed up healing of bruises. It helps with digestive issues and hiccups. It also tones the spleen and liver.

It blends well with sandalwood, geranium, lavender and rose.

Frankincense

This oil is extracted from the resin of the Boswellia carteri tree. It is also referred to as Olibanum. It has a pleasant, woody aroma that is a bit spicy and camphoric.

During the ancient times, frankincense was used by Egyptians as a face mask and an offering to their Gods. Hebrews valued this oil highly and was even offered as a gift to the baby Jesus. It was also used to ward off evil spirits and to cleanse the sick. In aromatherapy, it is used to calm the mind and create inner peace, making it a favorite among those who are meditating and doing yoga. It calms obsessive states and anxiety. It is also used during labor due to its calming effect. It also helps relieve rheumatism and boosts the urinary tract. It is also beneficial for rejuvenating the skin and helps heal wounds, carbuncles, skin inflammation and scars.

It blends well with bergamot, benzoin, lavender, lemon, pine, myrrh, orange and sandalwood.

Geranium

This oil is extracted from the leaves and stalk of the plant. This plant has approximately 700 varieties and only a few yield a good amount of oil. In the ancient times, Geranium was planted around houses to keep bad spirits away.

In aromatherapy, Geranium is one of the essential oils that are widely used. It clears the mind and balances emotions and the hormonal system. It also stimulates the lymphatic system and the adrenal cortex. It also keeps the skin supple while balancing sebum production to prevent acne. It is also beneficial for wounds, cuts, dermatitis and eczema. It also repels lice, mosquitos and ringworms. It is also used to cure breast engorgement, poor circulation, and PMS.

It blends well with angelica, basil, bergamot, carrot seed, citronella, cedarwood, clary sage, jasmine, grapefruit, lime, lavender, orange, neroli and rosemary.

Grapefruit

This essential oil is extracted from fresh fruit peels that are cold compressed.

Grapefruit tree is originally from Asia and is now cultivated in Israel, Brazil and the USA.

It has a strong uplifting effect, making it effective for counteracting stress, depression, fatigue and stiffness. It is also a diuretic, helping the body flush out toxins and get rid of cellulites. It also helps treat oily skin and acne and promotes hair growth.

It blends well with bergamot, geranium, frankincense, lavender and Palma Rosa.

Jasmine

This essential oil is obtained from the flowers of the evergreen shrub which originated in Northern India and China. For best results, the flowers are picked during the night as its aroma is at peak during this time.

It soothes the nerves and is an effective remedy for depression. The sweet, flowery, exotic aroma of this oil produces a feeling of euphoria, optimism and confidence. It also revitalizes and restores lost energy. It is also beneficial for treating post natal depression and supports better milk production. It also helps relieve respiratory ailments and muscle pains. It increases the skin's elasticity which helps reduce stretch marks and scarring.

It blends well with bergamot, citrus oil, sandalwood and rose.

Lavender

It is obtained from the flowering tops of the evergreen shrub known as English lavender, common lavender or garden lavender. The fresh, light smell of Lavender calms the mind and relaxes the body, which makes it great in relieving stress and anxiety and in combating crisis.

Its antiseptic properties help relieve flu, fever, colds, bronchitis, asthma, whooping cough and even throat infections and halitosis. It also helps relieve muscular and joint pains and is beneficial for all types of skin conditions. It is also an excellent insect repellant.

It blends well with clary sage, cedarwood, pine, geranium, all citrus oils and nutmeg.

Lemon

This oil is extracted from fresh fruit peels through cold expression. The sharp, fresh, citrus aroma of lemon helps improve concentration and supports better decision making. In Japan, banks use lemon essential oil in diffusers to help minimize worker-related errors. It is also a popular flavoring for food and as fragrance for perfumes.

In the Middle Ages, an ounce of lemon is given to the Royal Navy each day to treat vitamin deficiencies including scurvy. It is helpful for nosebleeds as it reduces blood pressure. It also helps lower fever, treat flu, bronchitis, asthma and throat infections.It also relieves migraines, headaches, insect bites and herpes. It's antiseptic and antibacterial properties help clear the skin and get rid of acne. It also removes excess grease from the skin and hair.

It blends well with benzoin, elemi, eucalyptus, fennel, geranium, juniper, lavender, rose, sandalwood and neroli.

Marjoram

It is extracted from the leaves and flowering tops of the bushy, perennial herb known as knotted marjoram. In ancient Greece, it was given to newlyweds as a token for good fortune. It was also widely used by the Greeks as medicine and perfume.

The warm, somewhat spicy aroma of this oil calms the emotions as well as tames hyperactive people. It releases stress and relieves anxiety. It also relaxes the muscles making it effective for muscle pains, spasms, strains and sprains. It also soothes the digestive system and relieves conditions associated to it. It also helps with insomnia, migraines and headaches. Take note that marjoram can reduce sexual desire.

It blends well with chamomile, cedarwood, cypress, eucalyptus, bergamot, tea tree and lavender.

Neroli

This oil is obtained from the flower of the bitter-orange tree known as orange blossom, orange flower or neroli bigarade. Its sweet, sharp floral smell has a great relaxing effect on the mind and body. It calms heart palpitations, treats depression, shock, and anxiety.

It helps treat diarrhea, colitis and spasm. It is very useful for the skin as it rejuvenates and regenerates skin cells. It prevents scarring, helps minimize stretch marks, treats broken capillaries, and supports smoother skin.

It blends well with lavender, geranium, jasmine, benzoin, ylang-ylang, sandalwood, rosemary and all citrus oils.

Rosemary

This is extracted from the flowering tops of the shrubby evergreen bush through steam distillation. During the Middle Ages, rosemary was used to keep away bad spirits. It's clear, refreshing herbal aroma promotes mental clarity, improves memory and stimulates the brain.

It also helps treat jaundice and relieves muscular and joint pains. It also helps reduce water retention and aids in weight loss and cellulite removal. It is popularly used for hair growth and hair and scalp care as it increases circulation to the scalp, stimulating growth and health.

It blends well with citronella, cedarwood, lavender, lemongrass, geranium and peppermint.

Sandalwood

It is extracted from the heartwood of the tree and has an exotic, lingering woody aroma that calms the mind and produces a harmonizing effect. It also reduces tension and confusion, fear, anxiety, stress and chronic illnesses.

It is also useful for chest issues, urinary tract problems, bladder infections as well as impotence and frigidity. It is also great for skin care as it tones the skin, relieves inflammation and itching, prevents scarring and fights eczema.

It blends well with myrrh, vetiver, rose, ylang-ylang, bergamot, geranium, black pepper and lavender.

Chapter 11: All About Essential Oils

The use of essential oils dates back to ancient times. Egyptians used them in their embalming process as well as using them in their cosmetics and burning of incense that contained essential oils.They used aromatic herbs for religious, medicinal, and aromatherapy purposes.They have also been used for centuries for their medicinal properties in folk medicine since ancient times much of which is still being used the same way today.

The term "essential oils" is derived from the term "quintessential oil."This originates from the Aristotelian thought or idea that matter was made from four elements those being fire, water, earth, and air.The life force or spirit of the plant was considered to be the fifth element or quintessence.During the process of distillation and evaporation was the time thought to be when the "spirits" were removed from the plants. Today we know that essential oils are physical in nature and are made up of a complex mixture of chemicals.

Essential Oils are a type of concentrated hydrophobic liquids which contain aroma compounds from the plants that they are extracted from through various forms of extraction.Other names that essential oils are known under are volatile oils, ethereal oils, aetherola or plainly"oil of" the plant that they were extracted from.Oils are known as essential because they have the scent of the plant that they come from.Essential oils are not essential for health, but many use them for medicinal purposes especially when using alternative medicine.

Today distillation is the most common process for collecting essential oil as it is easy to separate the condensed water.During the process, the plants are placed inside the still on the grid.The still is then sealed shut.Depending on the distillation process steam or water, the steam goes through the plant material removing the volatile constituents.These rise and go through a connecting pipe that takes them to the condenser.The condenser then cools the vapor back into a liquid form.There is a collection container below the condenser that collects the liquid.The water and essential oils do not mix, so the essential oils are collected from the top by a siphoning method.Sometimes the essential oils are heavier than the water in this case they are collected from the bottom of the liquid collector.Described below is an overview of the different processes.

Water Distillation:

This is an extraction method in which the plant material comes into direct contact with the water.This method is commonly used with flowers and orange blossoms as direct steam causes these to clump together making it difficult for steam to pass through.

Water and Steam:

This is employed with herb and leaf material the water remains below the plant material during this process; the steam comes from outside the main still indirectly.

Steam Distillation:

This is the most commonly used process of extraction; the steam is injected into still usually at a higher pressure and temperature than the above 2 methods.

Percolation:

This is the most recent method it is similar to steam distillation but instead of the steam coming in the bottom of still it comes through the top.This form of extraction makes for a shorter distillation time.It works very well when extracting essential oils from tough materials such as wood.

Expression (Cold Press):

This method is usually used in gathering citrus essential oils where the peels are pressed usually by mechanical machines to extract the essential oils from the citrus fruit skins.

Listed below are some essential oils, their benefits and some uses

Olive Essential Oil

• Good for Heart Health

- Full of monounsaturated fatty acids
- Olive oil may actually reduce your risk of heart disease by lowering cholesterol

Argan Oil

- Argan oil has been a beauty remedy for centuries
- This oil is perfect for multi-tasking
- Helps with brittle nails
- Good to apply to rough dry skin

Rosehip Oil

- Powerful exfoliant
- Full of vitamin E
- Will help to brighten and revive your skin
- Rosehip contains essential fatty acids which may improve dry skin conditions such as eczema and psoriasis

Lavender Oil

- For stress release
- Smelling lavender may reduce stress hormones in your blood
- Can help you rest/sleep at night (try putting some oil on your pillow)
- Good for dry and scaly skin

Manuka Oil

- Has anti-fungal properties

- May promote healing on cuts and scrapes

Peppermint Oil
- May ease symptoms of irritable bowel syndrome
- Can be ingested
- Mix small amount with water to help with indigestion

Lemon Essential Oil
- Lemons have many stress reducing properties which are concentrated in the oil
- Use lemon spray to help you to relax after a hard day at work
- Grate lemon peel and fill bottle half-way with rinds and the other half with oil let sit on window-sill for a few days great to use to help keep you in a calm state by smelling

Oil of Oregano
- Is one of nature's most powerful antibiotics
- Is effective in killing bacteria
- Can help the immune system to take action against fungi, viruses, and parasites

- Contains compound Carvacrolthat is known to break through the outer membrane that helps to protect bacteria from the immune system.

Safe Use of Essential Oils:

Make sure that you know how to properly apply the particular essential oil that you wish to use; they are not all applied or can be used in the same manner.Taking these precautions will help you to avoid any serious side effects.

Your risks will be minimal if you use essential oils in a proper and responsible manner. Essential oils that are sold for domestic or professional use are mostly safe.If you follow the basic guidelines and instructions, you should have no problems when using essential oils.You may get a minor skin irritation but nothing life threatening.

Guidelines to follow

Always use pure essential oils. There is an increased chance of experiencing an adverse side effect when using adulterated product; it is important to use pure essential oils.

Diluting with other oils

Some essential oils such as citrus based oils may cause irritation to skin if not diluted first with another carrier oil such as olive oil. Any oils that contain eugenol or cinnamaldehyde such as citrus or citronella, or cinnamon should be diluted before using on skin.

Ways to apply essential oils:

You can apply essential oils by taking them internally, diffuse them, inhaling, and on the skin. Each form of application has safety issues that must be addressed.

1) Skin application

You should avoid applying oils to damaged skin as the opening or wound will absorb more oils than normal which could cause you to absorb unsafe levels of essential oils. Try not to overuse essential oils on the skin as this could cause irritation to the skin.

Essential oils that may irritate skin are: Bay, Tagetes, Thyme, Oregano, Clove Bud, Lemongrass, Cinnamon bark, and Cumin

2) Diffusion

This is a form of dispersing the essential oils into the air so that their aroma fills the room with the natural fragrance of the essential oils. This method of application can be done through using a nebulizer or through the use of incense.Other types of diffusion methods are steam, simple tissue diffusion, candle, lamp ring, sandstone and terracotta diffusers.The earliest recorded use of this method was by the Andalusian physician, chemist, pharmacistIbn al-Baitar (1188-1248).

3)Internal ingestion

Most essential oils cannot be taken internally, so it is very important to make sure that you follow the instructions for taking essential oils internally.Some examples of these are peppermint, lemon and lavender oils.

4)Inhaling

There is no need to worry when inhaling essential oils in a small closed room; however proper instructions should always be followed.

Chapter 12: How To Use Essential Oils

Essential oils can be utilized in a thousands of different ways. The most common are listed below to help better understand the rest of the content in this lifestyle guide.

Diffusers

Passive diffusers - a diffuser that allows essential oils to be exposed to air so that the oils naturally evaporate and are dispersed into the air. Placing several drops of oil onto a tissue is one of the simplest methods of passive diffusion. Some of the more common commercial passive diffusers include terra cotta and ceramic diffusers.

Fan diffusers - devices that use a small fan which creates airflow over a pad or wick with the essential oils to disperse oils into the air.

Heat diffusers - heat diffusers, such as lamp rings, candle diffusers and electric heat diffusers, heat the essential oil to promote diffusion into the room.

Mist diffusers - mix water and essential oils together which then enter the surrounding air.

Nebulizers - nebulizers break the essential oils into tiny droplets.

Candle Work

You can rub a candle down with an essential oil or add a few drops to the crown of the candle before lighting. Avoid the wick, you don't want to start a fire.

Spiritual Baths

Add an appropriate number of drops to baths to be taken for relaxation or spiritual purposes.

Definitions

Aromatherapy - The science of utilizing naturally extracted aromatic essences from plants to balance, harmonize and promote the health of body, mind and spirit.It seeks to unify physiological, psychological and spiritual processes to enhance an individual's innate healing process

Essential Oil - Any of a class of volatile oils obtained from plants,

possessing the odor and other characteristic
properties of
the plant, used chiefly in the manufacture of perfumes, flavors, and pharmaceuticals.

Lavender Essential Oil

Name: **Lavender**

Scientific Name: Lavandula anguvstifolia **and** Lavandula officinalis

Expense: Average Price is $15 for 1 ounce of organic lavender oil

Essential oils have seen a noted increase in demand as knowledge of aromatherapy and holistic medical treatment have become more readily available to the public. Lavender is the most common, well known and easily accessible of the nearly infinite list of beneficial essential oils. Derived by distillation of the flower spikes on select species, this fragrant and healing oil has many benefits.

Lavender essential oil has been recorded helping humanity for more than 2,500 years, with Egyptians, Phoenicians and several other cultures using the oil for processes from the sacred right of mummification to a cure for insomnia. Even Romans values lavender as a prized commodity, often costing more than 100 denarii (the most common measure of roman currency) per pound. Used to scent bath houses, insect repellent and even flavoring, it was equivalent to one month's wages of a farm worker.

During the Renaissance, lavender was swept over the cold, damp floors of castles as both a deodorant and a disinfectant, as well as enjoying popular use in apothecaries gardens. The lavender flower saw another spike in popularity during the plague, where it became custom to adhere small bunches to each wrist as protection of the greatly feared Black Death. Once more its ability to repel insects helped stave off disease and pestilence.

In more recent history, the flower has more scientifically proven effects. Its use as a bug repellent remains as true in the current century, as it did thousands of years ago; with several studies proving it repels mosquitoes, midges, as well as most species of moth. Also, should one encounter a biting insect that is not put off by the oil, lavender has anti-inflammatory qualities that will reduce the irritation pain that often come hand in hand with biting insects.

However, this versatile plant's uses go far beyond its ability to dissuade pests. Lavender still continues to be used regularly as a treatment for insomnia. Many studies on elderly patients have showed an increase in regulation of their sleep cycles after the essential oil replaced their prescribed sleeping medication. It is widely believed in the scientific community that this is due to the flower's effect on the nervous system. Lavender regulates the heart-rate while also increasing cognitive function, creating the perfect combination of clarity of thought as well as relieving stress. This sympathetic reaction has also proven helpful in treating migraines, head aches as well as nervous and emotional stress without all the harmful chemicals of most modern over the counter remedies.

This neurological effect also allows the oil to be used as an efficient remedy for various bodily aches and pains, including sore or tense muscles, rheumatism, sprains and even strains. A massage with lavender essential oil can also provide relief from chronic joint pain. A study done on post-operative pain relief found that combining lavender oil vapor into the breathing masks of patients significantly reduced the amount of pain experienced, versus the patients that were revived with pure oxygen after their procedure.

This breath-mask study lead to other discoveries of lavender's ability to treat various respiratory problems, from throat infections, flu, colds, asthma, sinus congestion, bronchitis, whooping cough, laryngitis, and even tonsillitis. The oil can be use either in the form of a liquid that is applied on the skin of the neck, chest or back, or it can be added to vaporizers or inhalers that are commonly used for colds and coughs. The stimulating nature of lavender essential oil can also break up phlegm trapped within the respiratory system and relieve the congestion associated with breathing conditions. This increase of oxygen as well as the expulsion of germ-housing phlegm, can speed up the recovery process and help the body naturally eliminate other unwanted materials. The vapor of lavender essential oil also been found to have anti-bacterial effect which can battle respiratory tract infections.

Continuing with its hormonal benefits, Lavender essential oil is incredibly useful for treating urinary disorders, as it stimulates urine production while also restoring hormonal balance. It also has been found to reduce cystitis or inflammation of the bladder in both sexes, as well as relieving cramps in females.

However, Lavender essential oil's benefits are not purely internal. Both dermatologists and aromatherapists have listed the flower as one of the most beneficial oils for treating acne by regulating some of the over-excretion of sebum by hormonal manipulation. Adding a small amount of lavender essential oil to you daily regimen can prevent acne, as well as heal and prevent long term scarring.

Lavender's use in the beauty industry is not limited to removing blemishes. This essential oil is often used for nature-inspired hair care, as it has been shown to effectively neutralizer lice, lice eggs, and nits. Furthermore, lavender oil can be very helpful in the treatment of hair loss, particularly for patients who suffer from Alopecia, (an autoimmune disease where the body rejects its own hair follicles). According to a Sottish study "more than 40% of Alopecia patients reported an increase in hair growth when they regularly rubbed lavender essential oil into their scalp."

The list of physical benefits actually goes on further, including aiding digestion, preventing cancer and leucorrhoea. The only thing that may outnumber the uses of lavender essential oil is how to apply the treatment. The easiest, and most readily available way to utilize the oil is to rub two to three drops into your cupped palms then slowly and deeply inhale. This pulls the scent all the way to the amygdala gland for an expedient calming effect on the body. Another way is to rub a small amount onto the temples, wrists and feet.

More involved is the use of a diffuser, which disperses essential oils in the air to be breathed in naturally by breaking the liquid down into micro-molecules. Variants include ultrasonic, cold air, evaporator and heat diffusers. Prices on these small machines vary by area and brand. The best way to secure one is to either visit your local holistic outlet or shop online.

And perhaps the most common use is via aromatherapy during massage. The oil is mixed throughout the massage therapist's lotion and used during the session, applying the healing treatment over all of the skin.

Chapter 13: Diy Non-Toxic Cleaning Products

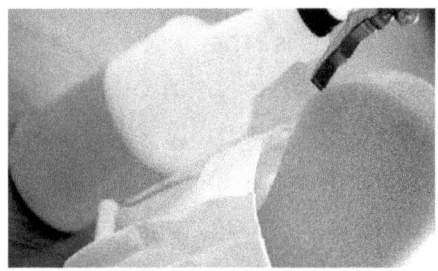

Toxins pose great threats to your health and the environment. Since you are reading this eBook, you want superior choices for yourself, your family and your home.

You made a wise decision. You do have reason for concern and many people are not aware of how dangerous many of these products are in beauty and cleaning products. Naturally, manufacturers want to sell their products, but at what cost to human health and the environment?

Reading the label on products sold in the store is no guarantee that what is in them isn't dangerous. Labels only warn you about the health hazards associated with a single or short-term exposure to chemicals in the product. No one knows the long-term consequences.

For beauty products and cleaning products you use often, this is very troubling. These chemicals absorb through your skin and traces of them stay on surfaces and end up in our water system too. They affect every living creature, including your household pets.

U.S. researchers tested six major commercial brands of all-purpose cleaners and every product had between one and eight toxic or hazardous chemicals in them as defined by U.S. law.

By and large, the beauty industry and cleaning products are unregulated. These industries self-monitor and pull products off the market when disaster strikes. They don't want you to know that they choose to use chemicals because they are cheap and they can make a profit, instead of focusing on your health.

They also spend millions of dollars to convince you that their new product is superior to what you could make yourself. This is not true. This eBook offers many recipes to prove to you that you can live without these harmful chemicals, have a healthier household and save money too. Try a few of them out and once you see how well they work you will want to eliminate the dangerous chemicals from your house once and for all.

Thanks to a few basic ingredients and your essential oils you can make countless beauty and household products, and at a fraction of the cost that you pay for the multitude of store-bought products in your cupboards now.

Join the green revolution. It's a wise choice.

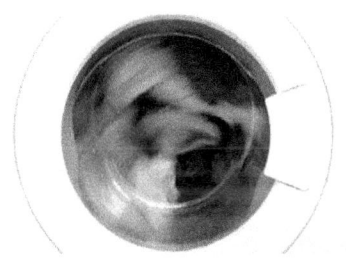

Homemade Laundry Detergent (powder)
1 cup washing soda
1 cup baking soda
1cup borax
1 bar of soap (Dr. Bronner's castile soap or any all natural bar soap of your choice)
1/2 cup all natural laundry whitener
10-15 drops of your favorite essential oil or combination (lavender, lemon, lime)
Sealable container
Run bar of soap through your food processor grater attachment. Add all other ingredients except oil and blend until soap and powders all thoroughly mixed (about 20-30 seconds). Add your essential oils and blend for another 20-30 seconds. Transfer to sealable jar or container and use 1-2 tbsp. per load.
Homemade Fabric Softener (for the dryer)

4 or 5 cut up J-clothes or sponges (can use old t-shirts, dish clothes, tea towels)
2 cups vinegar
20-30 drops of your favorite essential oil
Sealable container
Place rags in jar or container add vinegar and essential oils. Wring out one rag and add to your load in the dryer. When clothes are dry, simply put rag back into the sealed container.
Fabric Softener (washing machine)

Vinegar
Essential oil of your choice
Small pourable container

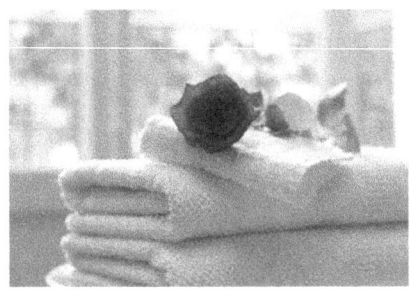

Fill container with vinegar and add 10-20 drops of favourite essential oil. Add to your fabric softener dispenser of your washing machine.

All Purpose Cleaner #1

Vinegar

Lemon Essential Oil or Tea Tree Essential Oil

Spray Bottle

Fill spray bottle with vinegar and 10-20 drops of essential oil into spray bottle. Use this to clean bathrooms, kitchens and any surfaces.

All Purpose Cleaner #2

1/4 cup vinegar

1 tsp borax

Warm water

2 tbsp. unscented Castile soap

10-15 drops of essential oils (lemon or tea tree)

Pour vinegar and borax into spray bottle.Swirl until dissolved. Fill bottle with warm water and shake. Add castile soap and essential oils and shake.

Homemade Room Spray

Empty spray bottle

1 tbsp. baking soda

2 cups distilled water

10 drops of essential oil (sweet orange is nice!)

Homemade Carpet Freshener

2 cups baking soda

10-20 drops essential oils

Shakeable sealable container (I use an empty parmesan cheese shaker)

Mix baking soda and oils together in container. Sprinkle on carpet or other fabrics, let sit for 10 or 20 minutes then vacuum.

Homemade "Comet"

2 cups baking soda

½ cup Borax

5-10 tea tree and lemon essential oil

Mix ingredients together in bowl and pour into an empty parmesan cheese shaker.

Glass & Mirror Cleaner

1/4 cup vinegar

1/4 cup rubbing alcohol

1 tbsp. cornstarch (reduces streaking)

8-10 drops essential oil

Mix all ingredients in spray bottle. Shake well before each use.

Toilet Bowl Cleaner
1/2 cup baking soda
1/4 cup castile soap
1/4 cup hydrogen peroxide
1 cup hot water
1/4 cup vinegar
10 drops of essential oil
Mix baking soda and castile soap together. Add peroxide and oils. Slowly add hot water. Stir in vinegar and stir until foaming stops. Pour into squeeze top bottle. Squeeze around inside rim of toilet bowl and let sit for 10 minutes before scrubbing with toilet brush.

Shower Spray
1 cup vinegar
1 cup castile soap
1 cup water
10-15 drops of essential oil
Mix all ingredients in spray bottle. After giving your shower a thorough scrubbing with your homemade "comet", use this spray daily after each shower.

Bug Repellant
1/2 cup witch hazel
8 drops of citronella

8 drops of lemongrass
6 drops of lavender
Put in spray bottle and shake.

Chapter 14: What Are Essential Oils?

Essential oils are the fragrant, natural constituents of plants. They give the plant its characteristic smell and also contain its healing power when extracted. They can bring a wide range of health benefits if used correctly and unlike modern drugs, they have zero side effects. A typical essential oil consists more than 100 chemical compounds, each of which has therapeutic use for a specific treatment. For this reason, many essential oils can be used for the treatment of a wide range of medical conditions. Almost all essential oils possess antiseptic properties, while many of them are also proven to have antifungal, antiviral and antibacterial properties.

A Brief History of Essential Oils

The use of essential, or aromatic oils as they were once called, can be traced back in history for thousands of years. Their usage varied between cultures and ranged from religious purposes to healing the sick.

The earliest evidence of human discovery about the plants' healing properties can be found in the Dordogne region of France. Cave paintings that suggest the use of medicinal plants in everyday life have been found that are dated as far back as 18000 BC.

Egypt

Evidence and recorded history have shown that in Ancient Egypt, people used aromatic oils as early as 4500 BC. The Egyptians became renowned for their knowledge of cosmetology and aromatic oils. The herbal preparation called "Kyphi" was a mixture of 16 ingredients that could be used as medicine, perfume, and frankincense.

The use of balsams, perfumed oils, scented barks, spices, resins and aromatic vinegar in everyday life has been well documented in the Egyptian history. They transformed oils and pastes from plants into pills, powders, medicinal cakes and ointments. At the peak of Egypt's power, the use of essential oils was only allowed to priests as they were regarded as necessary to be at one with the gods.

Specific fragrances were dedicated to each divinity. Their followers anointed each deity's statue with a mixture of these oils. There were also special mixtures and blends for Pharaohs, not only to support them in certain aspects in life, such as love, meditation, and war, but also for embalming their corpses once they were deceased. Traces of aromatic gums such as cedar and myrrh have been found on mummies today. Cedar essential oil was by far the most commonly used aromatic oil by ancient Egyptians. However, despite the importance of those oils in Egyptian society, they never distilled it themselves. In fact, they imported oils of cypress and cedar.

China

Historical records have shown that the use of aromatic oils in China goes back to 2697 BC during the reign of Huang Ti, the legendary Yellow Emperor. He documented the use of several aromatics in "The Yellow Emperor's Book of Internal

Medicine," which is still considered a useful classic by practitioners of eastern medicine today.

India

The use of essential oils in the traditional Indian medicine called "Ayurveda" has a 3000-year old history. Ayurvedic literature comprises over 700 substances including ginger, cinnamon, myrrh and sandalwood as effective for healing. The Ayurvedic approach of using those essential oils was successfully used in replacing ineffective antibiotics during the outbreak of the Bubonic Plague. What's more? The purpose of aromatic plants and oils was also believed to be a godly part of nature und shaped the spiritual and philosophical aspect in Ayurvedic medicine.

Greece

There is recorded knowledge about the use of essential oils in ancient Greece that reaches back to 400-500 BC. Greek soldiers carried ointment of Myrrh into battle to treat infections. The Greek physician Hypocrites, who is known as the

"Father of Medicine" documented the effects of more than 300 plants.

His extensive knowledge of plants had its origin in Ayurvedic medicine and was gained when Greek soldiers passed through India during their travels with Alexander the Great. Ayurveda was found to be harmonious with their own medicinal practices. There's also evidence of the mingling of these two traditions, which can still be found in use by remote tribes today.

In his literature, Hypocrites stated that "a daily perfumed bath and a scented massage is the way to good health." He further emphasized that the main purpose of a doctor is to awaken the natural healing abilities within the body.

Rome

It is well known that the Romans not only applied perfumed oil to their bodies, bedding, and clothes, but also put it to use for massage and baths.

Persia

The famous Ali-Ibn Sana, who became a well-educated physician by the age of 12, has documented the properties of 800 plants and their effects in his books. He is also assumed as being the first person to discover and record the method of distilling essential oils. Some of these methods are still in use today.

Europe

During the Crusades, the Knights and their armies learned a lot about essential oils and herbal medicines in the Middle East, including knowledge about distillation. They passed this knowledge throughout Western Europe on their return.

During his research of essential oils, French chemist René-Maurice Gattefossé minted the term "Aromatherapie." His book "Aromatherapie" was published in 1928. It described detailed cases of essential oils and their healing capabilities and was influential in medical practices in France.

He also discovered the healing properties of Lavender by accident. During a small explosion in his laboratory, one of his hands was burned badly. He quickly immersed it in the nearest tray of liquid, which turned out to be the essential oil of Lavender. To his surprise, Gattefossé observed that his hand healed without any signs of infection or scarring. After further research on lavender's healing properties, Gattefossé and a colleague introduced it to many French hospitals. There were no reported deaths of French hospital personnel, during the outbreak of the Spanish flu, which was credited to the use of lavender.

Chapter 15: The Power Of Smell

Did you know that our perceptions of each other are partly based on our personal aroma, not just our physical appearance or our behavior or ability to communicate? This is not just a theory. Research has proven repeatedly that we all have our own unique scent (though most of the time we are unaware of it) which can make us 'look' more appealing or otherwise to people around us. Our personal smell transmits information about ourselves, information that is subconsciously interpreted by others. Contrary to modern day advertisements, our personal 'base' smell cannot be altered with perfumes, aftershaves, deodorants, or fragrant body washes; at the most we may able to mask it temporarily.

Smells are important in many industries - perfumery, wine-making, coffee roasting, food-production, cosmetics and tobacco to list some of the more obvious ones.The perception of smell consists not only of the sensation of the odors themselves but of the experiences and emotions associated with these sensations. There exists a close relationship between scents, emotion and memories.Smell sensations are relayed to the cortex, where 'cognitive' recognition occurs, after the deepest parts of our brains have been stimulated. Thus, by the time we correctly name a particular scent as, for example, 'vanilla', the scent has already activated the limbic system, triggering more deep-seated emotional responses and long term memories. That is why many people suddenly and vividly recall distant memories when exposed to certain scents - the perfume worn by their mother, for example, can remind them of childhood.Certain aromas affect us psychologically; the smell of lemon is said to increase our perception of personal wellbeing.Supermarkets use the smell of freshly baked bread to make us feel hungry and buy more food, the smell of frankincense incense in a church can help us to feel more relaxed and in touch with our spiritual side.

Aroma means scent, and therapy means treatment. **Aromatherapy**, therefore, is a cure using the power of scents. It is derived from the ancient practice of using natural plant essences to promote health and wellbeing. Natural essences are contained in various parts of the plant, including its flowers, leaves, roots, wood, seeds, fruit, and bark -in the form of **essential oils**(they are the plants 'essence' or aroma-producing oils). The essential oils carry concentrations of the plant's healing properties -- those same properties that traditional Western medicine utilizes in many drugs.

Aromatherapy deals with the application of those healing powers by using the pure essential oils obtained from a wide assortment of plants, which have been steam distilled or cold-pressed from flowers, fruit, bark and roots.

These oils are harvested very carefully from specific plant parts, like the flower, at specific times of the growing cycle. Potentially vast quantities of plant material is required to produce small quantities of essential oil. Approximately 150 kilograms of lavender is required to make one liter of lavender essential oil. For this reason essential oils can be expensive, but then only small quantities of such oils are required for therapeutic benefits.

Professional aroma therapists focus very specifically on the controlled use of essential oils to treat ailments and disease and to promote physical and emotional well-being. There are three different modes of action in the body: pharmacological, which affects the chemistry of the body; physiological, which affects the ability of the body to function and process; and psychological, which affects emotions and attitudes. These three modes interact continuously. Aromatherapy is so powerful because it affects all three modes:

Physiological impacts:

Almost all essential oils have antiseptic properties and are able to fight infections. They also ease a wide assortment of physical conditions, including burns, aches, pains, infections, high blood pressure, dissolve mucus and open nasal passages, aid digestion and promote blood circulation.

Pharmacological impacts:

They stimulate the immune system and hormone production like insulin

Psychological impacts:

Aromatherapy may promote relaxation and help relieve stress. Aromatherapy also acts on the central nervous system, relieving depression and anxiety, reducing stress, relaxing, uplifting, sedating or stimulating, restoring both physical and emotional wellbeing.

As research is increasingly showing, smells can impact on almost everything, from dreams and emotions, driving, stress and gambling, to pain, concentration, memory and romance. Let's explore some of the real life situations where aromatherapy has proven to be effective.

Insomnia and stress

According to a report from Maryland University, clinical trials have shown that the smell of lavender can help in insomnia, anxiety, stress, and post-operative pain." There is now scientific evidence to suggest that aromatherapy with lavender may slow the activity of the nervous system, improve sleep quality, promote relaxation, and lift mood in people suffering from sleep disorders," say the researchers. Chamomile, vanilla, coffee and roses have similar calming effects. A Thailand study showed the smell from roses reduces both breathing rate and blood pressure.

Aromatherapy can also have a considerable influence on our emotions. Sniffing clary sage, for example, can quell panic, while the fragrance released by peeling an orange can make you feel more optimistic. Since your mind strongly influences your health and is itself a powerful healing tool, it makes aromatherapy's potential even more exciting.

Dreams

Smelling pleasant aromas before sleep can lead to more positive dreams. Researches show that the emotional content of subsequent dreams was linked to the smell. Those who had the pleasant smell (like sandalwood or rose) had significantly more pleasant dreams than those who had no smell and the people exposed to the unpleasant smell (like sulphur) had the most negative dreams.

Concentration

Spraying the scent of lavender during factory tea breaks in Japan has been shown to improve post-break production. Athletes who sniffed peppermint ran faster and had better concentration than those who had no smell, while children performed better at tests when exposed to the aroma of fresh strawberries.

Memory

Smells are very powerful triggers of specific memories, and are used in therapy to help recover lost memories. Research at Toronto University shows that memories triggered by smells of rosemary and clary sage tend to be clearer, more intense and more emotional.

Spending

Smells can have an effect on what we buy, how much we spend, and even on what we gamble. In one study based at a Las Vegas casino, there was a near 50 per cent rise in money gambled when a pleasant scent was sprayed around slot machines. Researchers at Chicago University found that 84 per cent of shoppers found identical new shoes more attractive when they were displayed in a room with a pleasant aroma compared to one with no smell. They also valued the shoes at £10 more.

Almost all essential oils have multiple benefits, so having just a collection of half-dozen in hand will help you treat a wide range of common physical ailments and emotional problems – and that is the beauty of aromatherapy.

For instance,

Frankincense essential oil (commonly used to help combat stress) provides a warm and soothing aroma that can help to calm respiratory problems such as asthma.

Jasmine helps to lift your mood by relieving stress and depression. It has also been used as an aphrodisiac.

Bergamot essential oil, which has a sweet citrus fruity aroma can help relieve some symptoms of depression, aid digestion as well as to help reduce tense muscles.

There are literally hundreds of different essential oils on the market, many of them will help you to relax and handle your stressful situations in a much better manner. You may need to experiment to see which oils work best for you. While a whiff of lavender releases feel-good hormones, a hint of eucalyptus may improve your alertness.

Chapter 16: The Most Effective Essential Oils For Weight Loss And Recipes

This chapter will give you the information you need to start losing weight with the use of essential oils. There are three sections. The first section will discuss essential oils that can have an effect on your physical well-being. The second section will discuss essential oils that will help with your mental and emotional well-being. The third section will list other essential oils that you can investigate if needed. You will learn how to deal with stress and other issues that may affect how you view food. If you take this two-pronged approach, you will find great success with your weight loss efforts!

The Physical Side

This section will discuss essential oils that will help deal with the physical problems of weight loss, such as low metabolism, hunger pangs and cravings, and low energy levels. When you improve both of these, it will be easier to lose weight. Speeding up your metabolism enables it to burn more energy, meaning it will burn more fat. This section will also describe oils that help reduce food cravings. With the physical sensations of hunger removed, it is a much easier task to lose weight.

Grapefruit Essential Oil

Grapefruit essential oil has many healing benefits, including the ability to curb food cravings, helping to boost metabolism, helping to increase energy and endurance, and it can even help reduce the accumulation of abdominal fat in the body. It can do all these things because grapefruit oil contains a natural chemical compound called nootkatone, which stimulates an enzyme in the body called AMPK. The interaction between nootkatone and AMPK accelerates chemical reactions in the brain, muscles, and liver, which enables all the benefits listed above. It is also used to help control sugar cravings, so if you have difficulty resisting those donuts in the breakroom or a candy bar, grapefruit oil can do wonders for you. Many people have found great success with weight loss by using grapefruit oil.

There are a couple ways to use grapefruit oil. First, you can use it aromatically by diffusing it through your home in an oil diffuser. You can also inhale directly from a bottle or with the use of a cotton ball, as described earlier.

A simple way to use grapefruit oil topically is to make it into a topical cream. You can do this easily by mixing it into a one to one (1:1) ratio with jojoba oil. You can rub this mixture into sore muscles or on your abdomen to improve digestion.

Also, grapefruit oil is an essential oil that can be used safely internally, as long as the oil you purchase is 100 percent pure, therapeutic grade oil. To ingest this oil, it needs to contain ONLY grapefruit rind oil (the essential oil is derived from the rind). You can add a single drop to a glass of water and drink it or add a drop to honey or a smoothie.

You can also make a cellulite cream out of grapefruit oil. Follow this recipe to do so, then rub it on problem areas to help reduce cellulite buildup.

Total Time: 2 minutes
Serves: 30

Ingredients:
30 drops grapefruit essential oil
1 cup coconut oil
glass jar

Directions:
Mix grapefruit essential oil and coconut oil together. Store in a glass container. Rub into areas of cellulite for 5 minutes daily.

Make sure to be aware of the adverse effects of any essential oil. Grapefruit oil is considered safe, but it may interact with antidepressants and blood pressure medications. Also, if you are using it topically, stay out of the sun for at least one hour after application. Also, as always, make sure to apply the oil to a small portion of your skin before general use to make sure that you do not have any skin reactions. This is especially true if you have sensitive skin. You should do this with any topical application of any essential oil.

Lemon Essential Oil

Lemon essential oil has properties that can help both with the physical and the emotional aspects of weight loss. It has also been shown to have its properties enhanced when used in conjunction with grapefruit oil. These two oils used together can help with the breakdown of fats in the body, enhancing their weight loss properties.

The effects of lemon oil include suppressing weight gain, increasing energy, enhancing and improving mood, and as a pain reliever. When your mood is improved, people find it easier to stick to their weight loss plan. When negative feelings are dealt with, it is easier to stay positive and have more willpower, especially since many people struggle, more with overeating when they are in a bad mood. And with the physical effects of suppressing the body from storing fat, it has a two-pronged approach to weight loss.

Plus, if pain keeps you from exercising and staying active, lemon oil is a great pain reliever. And with the pain banished from your life, it is easier to establish an exercise routine and stick to it. By taking it after exercise, you can prevent pain from setting in.

To use lemon essential oil for weight loss, you can inhale it off a cotton ball or through a steam bath before you eat. This will help to reduce your appetite, so you eat less without being hungry and are able to lose weight easier. When lemon essential oil vapor is inhaled, it helps to stop you from overeating. Lemon oil, along with peppermint oil (see below), were the two scents that have been proven to prevent overeating and were the most effective in losing weight. These two oils are ones that you need to add to your arsenal!

To make a massage oil from lemon essential oil, add two drops to the carrier oil of your choice and massage it in where fat accumulates. A great carrier oil to use for all weight loss recipes, if not otherwise stated is coconut oil. This helps to eliminate toxins in the fat areas of the body, making them easier to burn.

To use this internally, just add two drops of food grade oil to your morning glass of water to help improve digestion and to eliminate toxins in the body. Again, make sure that your oil is of food grade if you plan on doing this.

To make a spray with lemon essential oil and other oils to spray in your room to promote relaxation, follow this recipe. When you are relaxed and not stressed out, it is easier to stick to your diet and not be tempted to eat to bring up your mood.

Room Spray

Ingredients:

6 drops eucalyptus essential oil
6 drops bergamot or lemon essential oil
4 drops pine essential oil
2 drop peppermint essential oil
2 ounces purified water

Instructions:
Combine oils and water in a glass spray bottle. Shake well and spray to combat odors and to promote a relaxing atmosphere.

Peppermint Essential Oil

There are several health benefits to peppermint essential oil, including increasing energy and mental alertness, it improves and elevates the mood, aids in digestion, and helps to reduce appetite. All these effects help you to stick to your diet, as you will be less hungry, food will move through your body faster, and you will have increased energy and mood, leading to a healthier, more active lifestyle without stress-induced eating that so many people suffer from.

Suppressing the appetite is one of the biggest draws of using peppermint essential oil. One study, completed in 2008, showed that people who inhaled peppermint essential oil every two hours reported that they did not feel hungry all the time and ate significantly fewer calories than people who did not inhale the oil. It is worthwhile to use this oil in a diffuser or on a cotton ball to suppress your appetite before every meal. Peppermint oil, along with lemon oil, were the two scents that proved to prevent overeating and were the most effective in losing weight. These two oils are ones that you need to add to your arsenal!

Besides inhaling it, peppermint essential oil is a great one to add to a bath. Add 5 to 10 drops to your morning bath to increase your energy for the day and to help suppress your appetite.

You can also take internally by adding one to two drops of the food grade, pure oil to reduce appetite and prevent overeating.

Peppermint oil should not as a topical application if you are pregnant or for children under the age of seven.

A good recipe utilizing peppermint oil, grapefruit oil, and lemon oil to help burn fat is to make a capsule from these oils. Use the recipe below to do so. You can buy capsules for essential oil use online or from any good purveyor of essential oils.

Fat-Burning Trio For Internal Use

Have one of these capsules every day after breakfast with a glass of water to help curb your appetite and speed up fat-burning mechanisms. Make sure to buy quality essential oils for internal use (food grade).

Ingredients (per capsule)
2 drops peppermint EO
2 drops grapefruit EO
2 drops lemon EO
12 drops coconut oil (liquefied)
Combine the ingredients in one capsule. You could multiply the recipe by mixing the EOs in an amber vial, add six drops of the mix into a capsule together with 12

drops liquefied coconut oil. Store pre-made capsules in the fridge for later use.

Cinnamon Essential Oil

Cinnamon oil has some great properties to help your body avoid weight gain. It improves insulin sensitivity, regulates blood sugar levels, and it reduces inflammation. To understand how it works, you need to understand a little bit about insulin. Insulin works in the body to metabolize carbohydrates and fat, which helps the body absorb blood glucose. It will either convert the carbs and fat to energy or store it. When fat cells in the body no longer respond to insulin, the body starts to store more fat instead of burning it, leading directly to weight gain. This also makes it harder to lose weight. Plus, this is the beginning of Type 2 diabetes. Cinnamon essential oil is used to help improve insulin sensitivity and increase the rate of blood glucose uptake, allowing for easier weight loss.

Cinnamon oil also helps to suppress the appetite and boosts metabolism. Between all these effects, cinnamon is one of the best oils to use for weight loss!

As with the other oils discussed, you can inhale a couple drops on a cotton ball before meals to reduce your appetite. You can also add it to a diffuser to decrease your appetite and make your home smell better.

To take internally, add one to two drops of food-grade cinnamon essential oil to a cup of warm water with a little honey in the morning, before a meal, or at night to avoid craving at night! A couple drops of cinnamon oil can also be added to other recipes to get the same effect. Just make sure that you don't add it to recipes that are cooked at a high temperature, as that can break down the active ingredients.

A good snack to make from cinnamon oil is below. This will help take away the munchies by utilizing cinnamon oil and satisfying that sweet tooth!

Crispy Cinnamon Baked Apple Chips

Recipe

Total Time: 1 hour

Serves: 7–8

Ingredients:
several large organic apples, about 7–8
1 tablespoon of your favorite natural sweetener, like raw honey or maple syrup of choice
6 drops pure cinnamon essential oil

Directions:
Preheat oven to 225 degrees F. Line 1–2 baking sheets with some parchment paper greased with coconut oil.
Thinly slice your apples using a mandolin or knife so they're about the same thickness. Toss the apples with sugar and oil, then add them to the baking sheet.
Bake them at no higher than 250 degrees for about one hour, flipping halfway through.

The main concern with cinnamon oil is that it may burn or cause pain when taken internally, especially if you have ulcers in your mouth. Also, this oil could have adverse effects if you have a heart problem, so check with your health care provider if you have any of these issues or you take any medication.

Fennel Essential Oil

Fennel oil is distilled from fennel seeds. It helps to improve digestion, suppresses the appetite, helps prevent the body from gaining more weight, and provides a more restful sleep. And if you sleep better, you are generally in a better mood, which helps curb overeating and emotional eating.

Fennel oil contains melatonin, a hormone that helps to regulate the body's circadian rhythms. In the body, melatonin reduces weight gain by helping the body create more of what is called beige fat, which is known to help burn energy. In the middle ages, fennel was used to help suppress the appetite on religious fasting days. A recent study showed that in laboratory rats, it did help suppress the appetite. Over an eight-week period, rats who inhaled the fennel essential oil twice a day for ten minutes each ate fewer calories and the food passed through the digestive tract faster. Both these things are linked with weight loss.

One way to fight cravings with fennel oil is to put a single drop of it under your tongue to help reduce sugar cravings. This is especially helpful if your weight loss efforts are sabotaged by a sweet tooth.

Inhale fennel seed oil twice a day off of a cotton ball as described previously or through a diffusor to suppress the appetite. The vapors also help you deal with stressful situations, keeping you calm. This will also help in your weight loss efforts.

To make a fennel lotion bar, combine ¼ cup each of coconut oil, almond oil, and beeswax (all carrier oils). Melt these together, then add ten drops each of fennel essential oil and lemon essential oil. Then, pour the mixture into a silicone mold and let it set for 24 hours before using it. This mixture will help keep your skin soft and smooth and is a good way to get the vapors on your body, which will help you suppress the appetite. The combination of the lemon and fennel oils works wonders for appetite suppression.

Emotional and Mental Issues

This section will list essential oils that will help you deal with the mental and emotional sides of weight loss. Depression, stress, anxiety, and general unhappiness will sabotage your weight loss efforts. They cause emotional food cravings, emotional eating, and lessens will power and the desire to stick to the diet as you have chosen. If you deal with these emotions in a healthy and effective way, you will naturally eat less because you won't be driven to make yourself feel better by eating foods that you shouldn't have or that you don't really want.

Bergamot Essential Oil

Bergamot essential oil helps to improve your energy level and boosts your mood. Anxiety and depression are two of the biggest causes of overeating. Of course, overeating will often lead to feeling worse than you did before, even if it gave you some immediate comfort. This starts a vicious cycle that is hard to stop.

But using bergamot oil can stop this vicious cycle. Studies have shown that people who inhale the bergamot oil for fifteen minutes a day reported feeling less stressed and a more positive mood. And we all know that in dieting, feeling good translates into making good food decisions.

To start, inhale the vapors of this oil through a diffuser, steam bath (as described earlier) or on a cotton ball for fifteen minutes a day to improve your mental and emotional health. Many people have reported that this is the perfect oil to inhale in your cranky days to feel better.

Another easy way to utilize bergamot oil is to dilute a few drops in a suitable carrier oil, such as olive oil or coconut oil. Then, use this to massage into your neck or your feet. Doing this in the morning will help to cut down on overeating and will help you deal more productively with negative emotions. You can also add a couple drops of bergamot oil into your morning bath to help you start the day on a positive note and set the tone for a happy day without emotional eating.

Last, the recipe below is a good way to add tension-reducing oils to your bath to help you relax.

Tension Tamer Bath Salt Recipe

Ingredients
2 cups Epsom Salt OR Dead Sea Salt
1 cup Sea Salt
1/2 cup Baking Soda
6 drops Bergamot essential oil
6 drops Sweet Orange essential oil
3 drops Lavender essential oil
Optional: 6 drops red, 4 drops yellow food coloring

Directions
Mix salt and baking soda together in a bowl using a metal spoon (a wooden

spoon will absorb the essential oils and be ruined.)

Drop in the essential oils and food coloring, placing each drop in its own little spot on top of the salts. Stir until thoroughly mixed.

Store mixture in a dark glass or PET plastic jar. Let cure at least 24 hours before using.

Use about one cup of salts per bath. This bath salt recipe makes enough for three baths.

Be careful with the topical application of bergamot oil, such as in the recipe above, as it can cause sunburn if you are exposed to direct sunlight after application. Also, do not use this oil if you are pregnant. It may cause irritation if you suffer from dry skin. It is also important to note that this is one oil that will degrade very quickly, so only buy it in small amounts that you will use in a short time. Make sure that you store it appropriately, as described above.

Lavender Essential Oil

Lavender essential oil is considered the one of the most essential of oils to use, and has a lot of wonderful effects for becoming more calm and relaxed. It helps to restore the nervous system, promotes sleep, increases inner peace, and helps you deal with panic attacks, anxiety, nervous tension, and even calms a nervous stomach. With all these positive emotional effects, it is one of the go-to oils to use to deal with stress and emotional eating. If you are anxious or depressed, this could be your best solution. Several studies have proven its stress-reducing capacities. If you are an emotional eater or eat when stressed out, you need to add this oil to your arsenal.

We will share with you a couple different recipes to make with the lavender essential oil. Because it is so versatile, it is worthwhile to have it on hand for many different things.

Lavender Bubble Bath

Store this in a bottle and keep it around to relax after a stressful day, instead of reaching for the ice cream!

2/3 c liquid glycerin

1 c clear, unscented dish soap

15+ drops lavender essential oil

Dried lavender {which will color your bubbles}

4 Tbsp. water

2 tsp salt

Gently mix in a mixing bowl and add to your container.

The next recipe is for a soothing sleep balm. If you have trouble sleeping, this may serve to help you out. And we all know that we are happier and healthier when we get enough sleep.

Ingredients needed:

1/4 cup Lemon balm

1/4 cup Chamomile flowers

Lavender essential oil

Vitamin e oil

1 1/2 cups Coconut oil (You can also use Jojoba oil, olive oil or grapeseed oil)

2 Tbsp. Candelilla wax or Beeswax (If using a liquid carrier oil instead, increase wax to 1/4 cup)

Directions:

Turn your oven on to 200 degrees, then turn it off. Combine coconut oil and herbs in an oven-proof pan/bowl. Stick the herbs & oil in the heated oven. Let them steep for about 3 hours. Use this time to play with your kids. They'll appreciate it.

Now, take out your herbs and strain the infused oil into a glass quart jar (or bowl). I really love those mesh strainers that fit into a bowl. You can toss the herbs once they've drained.

Clean out your pan and pour your strained oil into it. Put it back on the stove and turn it on to low heat. Stir in wax and let it melt. Turn off the heat and add 5 – 10 drops of lavender essential oil. Start low and if it doesn't smell strong enough, add more.

It's easy to overdo it with lavender, so add a few drops at a time. Then add 10 drops of the vitamin E oil. It helps to keep it from going rancid.

Pour your balm into dry (make sure they are very dry) jars, put the lid on and wait for it to dry. Make a nice label for your jar(s) so you can remember what's in there.

The third recipe is for an air freshener. To keep lavender in your home and to help keep everyone relaxed, here is a great recipe for an air freshener spray that you can use. The relaxing smell of lavender will keep you calm, relaxed, and away from the comfort food.

What you need:
2 cups water
1 tbsp. of baking soda
15-20 drops of therapeutic grade essential oil (depending on the strength of the oil you are using)
You can use just one scent (for example 20 drops of Lavender) or mix scents together (10 drops of Lavender and 10 drops of Chamomile).I prefer using a Lavender/Chamomile blend for bedrooms and a citrus blend of sorts for the kitchen and living room. The possibilities are endless!

Directions:

Pour the baking soda into a medium sized bowl. Drop the essential oil(s) over the baking soda and mix well. This will ensure that the oil is 'carried' in the powder and does not separate from the water.

Add the water and stir well until the baking soda has dissolved. Use a funnel and transfer into a spray bottle.

Spray away knowing that you are filling your home with natural safe scents!

Lastly, here is a simple recipe for a neck rub.

Easy Lavender Neck Rub

Ingredients:

3 drops pure lavender oil

1 teaspoon fractionated coconut oil or almond oil

Directions:

Blend the lavender oil and coconut or almond oil in your palm and rub onto your neck for natural anxiety relief. You can also rub onto the bottoms of your feet. This is perfect for anytime or just before bed.

If you don't have time to make any of the above recipes, you can always just drop two or three drops into your hands or on a cotton ball and inhale the scent when you are feeling stressed and need something to help you relax. If you are having trouble sleeping, rub a drop of lavender essential oil in your hand and then smooth it on your pillow to help you promote good sleep.

Lavender should do wonders for helping you deal with the mental and emotional issues that may cause you to overeat, eat emotionally, or to gain weight. If you have any of these problems, using lavender is an essential tool in your weight loss efforts.

Other Oils to Check Out

The oils listed in this chapter are some of the best and proven oils that you can use to promote the physical, mental, and emotional needs that you have when you are trying to lose weight. However, they are not the only ones that you can use. Once you have investigated some of these oils and incorporated their use in your dieting and weight loss efforts, there are some others you can check out and try.

Rose oil: This has been shown to be another great essential oil to help relieve depression and anxiety. A ten-minute inhalation and having your feet rubbed with rose oil can do wonders with relieving anxiety.

Vetiver oils: This oil offers grounding, tranquillity, and reassurance and helps deal with panic attacks. It also helps improve self-awareness.

Ylang Ylang oil: This oil was featured in one of the earlier recipes. It has been shown to elevate mood, optimism, and to sooth people when they feel fear. It can also help you sleep.

Essential oils that help to curb appetite: One of the biggest reasons that people fail at losing weight is that they cannot tolerate feeling hungry day after day after day. Some oils to check out for appetite suppression include any citrus oil, juniper, cypress, petitgrain bigarade, and black pepper.

Other oils to investigate: Tangerine, cloves, spearmint, ginger root, sandalwood, lemongrass, patchouli, celery seed, laurel, eucalyptus, hyssop, rose geranium, and ototea. These oils have been shown to help weight loss efforts in a variety of ways. If you are continuing your weight loss journey and want to add new oils, these are the ones to check out.

Chapter 17: Benefits Of Essential Oils

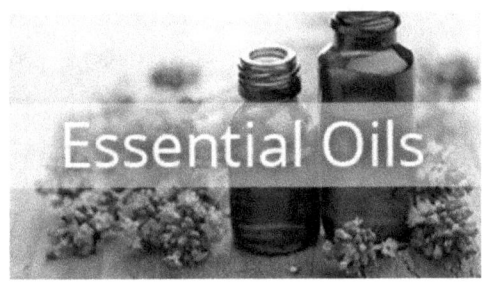

Essential oils contain numerous benefits and we are going to look at some of them.

Are able to penetrate your skin immediately

One of the benefits of essential oils is the fact that they are able to penetrate through your skin and cell membranes immediately. It only takes seconds for them to diffuse through your blood and tissues. These oils have the ability to get through the brain-blood barrier in order to get to the amygdale and various limbic parts of the brain. These are the parts that are in charge of controlling our mood, beliefs and emotions. This means that essential oils are capable of changing these three in order to enable us cope with stress, anger and the various emotions we are facing.

They have oxygenating properties

Essential oils contain oxygen molecules. They can therefore transport this oxygen to other cells in our bodies that are deprived of oxygen and to cells that need nutrients too. The cells in our body need oxygen to be healthy in order to be able to perform their functions properly and essential oils help with this.

They soothe muscles and joints

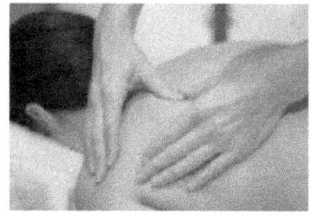

If you are suffering from aching muscles and joints then essential oils might be a good remedy for that. You may have minor aches and pains due to the everyday activities you engage in and essential oils can still help to take care of this. When you combine them with massage then you get even better results.

They contain high levels of antioxidants

Essential oils have been known to contain high level of antioxidants, which help the body. Antioxidants are responsible for strengthening your body's system. This enables the body to prevent negative effects that diet, aging and the environment have on our bodies. They also do away with free radicals. If you want to know the antioxidant capacity that essential oil contain then look at the ORAC (Oxygen Radical Absorbance Capacity) value indicated.For example clove essential oil's ORAC value is 1, 078, 700 µTE/100g. This is very high compared to the one for carrots, which is at 210 µTE/100g.

They soothe digestion

Essential oils have been known to soothe digestion. Peppermints also known as

Mentha Piperita are great herbs known for soothing digestions. They can also help to restore your digestive efficiency.

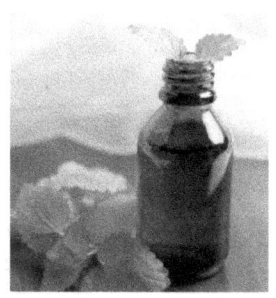

Are convenient and easy to use.
Essential oils are quite convenient in the sense that you can use them anywhere. Did you know that you could wear essential oils during the day? Yes, it is true and you can do this whether you are at home or work place. You can even carry them in your pocket. These oils are important in massage too and they can improve your level of meditation and concentration.

Can be used on animals too

It's amazing that the use of essential oils is not limited to humans. Animals have been known to respond well to these oils too and great examples are dogs and horses. Although there are some limitations when it comes to cats, they can still be used on them.

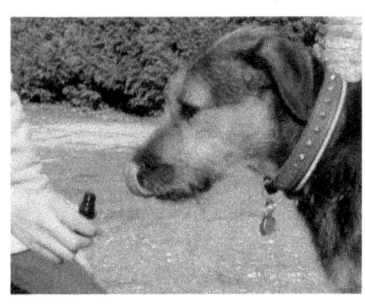

Are safe for use
Essential oils have the ability to restore your body's balance without harming it. This is due to the fact that they do not contain any chemical based products. However, ensure to choose therapeutic grade essential oils and not the perfume grade ones because the latter are made of up harmful chemicals.

Multi –purpose
There are essential oils that perform more than one function. For example, true

lavender essential oil also known, as Lavandula angustifolia is great for cuts and minor burns because it is gentle on the skin and contains antimicrobial properties too. It can also promote sleep and relaxation when inhaled. Therefore you don't need to buy lots of essential oils.
Essential oils refine your skin

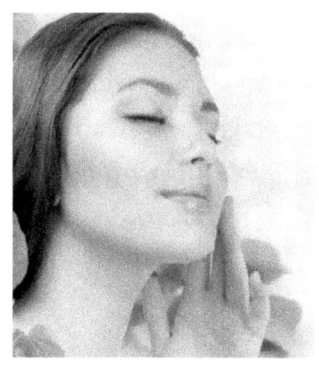

Using beauty products with lots of chemicals can sometimes diminish your natural glow. However, when you resort to essential oils then you can have it back. Essential oils help to give you a clear-looking complexion. In addition to that, they reduce the appearance of aging signs and give you healthy-looking hair.

Create deep spiritual awareness

Essential oils have always been used in both spiritual and religious ceremonies. They help people to connect with a higher being than themselves. According to research, these essential oils have compounds that stimulate olfactory receptors. If you want to enhance your spiritual experience then you can dilute the essential oils and apply them directly to your feet, wrists, behind the ears or let them diffuse in a quiet environment where you want to have your spiritual meditation.

Chapter 18: Essential Oils For Insect Bite And Repellent Spray

An insect bite is very painful. In some cases, insect bites are dangerous. You can have discomfort, swelling, pain, and itching. You can use medications to improve the condition and to prevent the spreading of the infection. But you cannot use these medications without a prescription. The process will be lengthy and will make the condition worse. But you can use essential oil blends to reduce the symptoms and to prevent the spreading of the infection.

Essential oil blend recipes for insect bites

1. For an insect bite

You can use essential oil blends to reduce the symptoms of an insect bite. For this blend, you will need 10 drops of Roman chamomile oil, 5 drops of peppermint oil, 12 drops of lavender oil, and 6 drops of lemon oil.

2. Insect repellent spray

If you have a lot of insects in your garden and you find it difficult to control them, you can use essential oil blends to control their spreading and to prevent their appearance. This blend will not affect your plants. It will also spread a pleasant aroma that you will not experience with the chemicals usually used to kill the insects in your garden. To prepare this blend, you will need 12 drops of rosemary oil, 10 drops of peppermint oil, 8 drops of clove oil, and 12 drops of thyme oil. All these essential oils are considered good to kill insects. But these are not harmful to humans. You can simply spray this blend on the soil to kill the insects or to prevent their appearance.

3. Bug repellent

Bugs are a common household problem. Many people have bugs in their home. They use different types of methods to get rid of the bugs permanently. But many of them do not offer a lasting solution. Even if they get relief for a temporary period, they do not get a permanent result. The bugs keep coming. If you are one of these people, you can consider using essential oils. This is an easy and simple method but offers an effective result. To make this blend, you will need 7 drops of lavender oil, 12 drops of lemongrass oil, 10 geranium oil, and 8 drops of peppermint oil.

4. For bacteria

If you want to kill the bacteria in your home and to make your living place more hygienic, you might need to spend a decent amount on chemicals every month. Moreover, these methods might not be healthy for your pet and your younger kids. If you are looking for a safe option and a lasting solution, you can use essential oils. For this blend, you will need 30 drops of clove oil, 25 drops of lemon oil, 5 drops of eucalyptus oil, 10 drops of cinnamon oil, and 3 drops of rosemary oil. You can use this blend to protect your home from bacteria and to kill them.

Essential oil blends offer different types of benefits. You can just simply take a drop of lavender oil on a cotton ball and can apply it on your skin directly to prevent mosquitoes. If you want to humidify your home, you can simply add 9 drops of tea tree oil. You can also use essential oils as a room freshener. You can use any of the essential oils of your preference. A few drops of oil will refresh the air and environment. Moreover, these are safe and will not cause any allergies. Even if you have breathing problems and you are allergic to the room freshener, you can use essential oils. These oils will not irritate you in any manner. You just need to choose the right essential oil and the blend to get the desired result.

Chapter 19: Types Of Essential Oils

This incredibly popular oil has all kinds of benefits. This subtly floral scent can help people to relax and sleep. Moreover, breathing it in has been found to help with alleviating headachesTrusted Source, while the use of the oil topically may help reduce the itching and swelling from bug bites.

Safety: There are a few known side effects. These include nausea, headaches, chills, and vomiting. It can also irritate the skin if you have an intolerance.

Roman chamomile

Featuring a combination of a light floral and herbal aroma, this oil has the potential to put your mind at ease when diffused and inhaled through steam. While this oil is great for calming the mind, it's equally as useful on the skin, and has been foundTrusted Source to treat conditions like inflammation and eczema.

Safety: Anyone allergic to daisies, marigolds, and ragweed should avoid using this oil altogether.

When the sweet, floral scent of rose oil is inhaled, it's been shown to help reduce anxiety. Its antioxidant properties have also been foundTrusted Source to help treat acne and improve complexion for an overall younger look.

Safety: Skin irritation can occur when used topically, so make sure to use more of the carrier oil if you want to reap the skin care benefits of rose oil.

This earthy, herbal, and sweet-scented essential oil can be used on the skin to help to minimize scarring, decrease inflammation, and act as an overall healing agent.

Safety: Don't use hyssop if you're pregnant or have a history of seizures.

This flowery oil emits a spicy but sweet aroma, and has been suggested as an aid in relaxation, a self-esteem builderTrusted Source, and it even may act as a repellant toward certain insects. It's frequently found in cosmetics and promises a laundry list of beauty benefits, including the treatment of combination skin and promotion of hair growth.

Myrrh

This sappy-smelling essential oil is said to treat skin issues by relieving acne and cracked skin, and may even help treat athlete's foot.

This spiced essential oil has antibacterial, antiviral, and antifungal benefits that may help treat athletes foot, bacterial infections, psoriasis, and warts. One studyTrusted Source found that it has strong antioxidant properties and could help treat fevers and respiratory symptoms, too.

Its sharp, spicy scent with hints of herbal tendencies can be used in aromatherapy, or applied topically to reap its benefits.

Safety: If you're pregnant or breastfeeding, you should talk to your doctor before using oregano oil.

Essential oil accessories

Once you've found the right essential oils for you, why not invest in a few accessories? From drawers to store your bottles and diffusers, to items to help you enjoy your essential oils on the go, there's plenty of items to choose from.

A drawer for your oils

If you find that your essential oil bottles are starting to take over too much counter space, an organizer of sorts is definitely in order. This box can act as a great way to keep track of all your bottles, while being a pretty addition to your home's décor.

Carrying case

Whether you only have a select few oils that you use on a daily basis, or find yourself traveling with a few you really love, this small bag will help keep up to 10 of them in place.

Mini diffuser

Ever need a bit of aromatherapy on the go? This oil diffuser plugs into your car so you can calm yourself on the way to a big meeting, or boost energy levels on the way to a dinner.

Ultrasonic diffuser

For those who don't want a big, bulky diffuser, this sleek white model is pleasing both aesthetically and therapeutically. Just plug it in and steam will emit in a beautiful light mist for all to enjoy.

Necklace

If you're someone who likes to take their aromatherapy everywhere they go, this cool, funky locket is exactly what you need. It comes in three shade rose gold, antique bronze, or silver with a replaceable pad of your essential oil choice on the inside.

Droppers and accessory bottles

For all those DIY types out there, these glass bottles are a great way to store the essential oils you love to use in your favorite recipes. The droppers make it so easy to measure, while the dark glass helps the oils keep their potency. Not to mention, they'll look amazing on any shelf. While there's still a good deal of research that needs to be done to fully back and support essential oils as a way to treat various health issues, there are still a number of benefits worth exploring.

Remember that essential oils must be diluted in a carrier oil before applying to the skin. Do not swallow essential oils. Some are toxic.

From alleviating insect bites to making your home smell great, essential oils offer a wide range of potential benefits.

Essential oils, which are obtained through mechanical pressing or distillation, are concentrated plant extracts that retain the natural smell and flavor of their source. Each essential oil has a unique composition of chemicals, and this variation affects the smell, absorption, and effects on the body. The chemical composition of an essential oil may vary within the same plant species, or from plant to plant. As an example of how concentrated essential oils are, 220 pounds of lavender flowers are required to produce approximately one pound of lavender oil. Synthetic oils are not considered true essential oils.

Chapter 20: The Power Of Nature: Dangers And Safety

Now that we know what essential oils actually are, where they come from, how they're used, and how the heck they have endured for all this time, I think it's time that we address something that will inevitably come up whenever you research essential oils, and that's the warning.

Before we go any farther than mentioning that, let me assure you that there are regulations and standards in place that are going to protect you from whatever you're afraid of. They're not going to bottle acid or pure nightshade and sell it to you.

However, these are raw, natural ingredients and in their highest potency, they can be very harmful to you. So it's important to address the dangers and the problems that could possibly face you if you abuse essential oils or if you go through the wrong connections.

This entire chapter is actually addressed to those that are looking to go really organic and want to buy from a local apothecary that someone has set up in an attempt to start a business. Innocent things can be deadly and it's important to have a healthy respect for what nature is capable of.

The first thing that you're going to want to know is that dilution is the solution to any problem that comes with the potency of essential oils. The
higher the level of purity, the more harmful they will be to you. So before you buy a bottle of cinnamon extract from a guy with a really long beard and a flannel shirt, make sure that he has listed purity and actually does his homework on it. You don't want to fry your skin. When an essential oil is far too potent for your body, it can cause severe problems, especially in sensitive areas just like your eyes or your mouth. While essential oils are either used for aromatherapy or for ingestion to alleviate symptoms of pain and congestion.

Another period in you life when you should not be taking essential oils is when you're pregnant. Essential oils are highly concentrated doses of plant essences, which is the aroma of a plant. If you know anything about pregnant women, you'll understand exactly where I'm going with this. Essential oils are potent smelling and if you want to make a pregnant woman try to kill you or banish you from their presence forever, bring something smelly around. Over all, I would advise you not to use essential oils if you are pregnant, plan to be, or have a pregnant woman around you. It's just common sense with this one.

If you're going to go the route from buying from a local apothecary, you need to do the research on what kind of a place that you're shopping from. One of the key things that you need to watch for is the quality of the original products that they're receiving.

You want to buy from apothecaries that have suppliers that are one hundred percent organic. The reason for this is that there are very harmful and very dangerous pesticides that are used to keep crops and vegetation free from insects that ravage crops. If you're not putting essential oils that are regulated and are completely organic, you risk the possibility of having poisons put on your body, inhaled, or in your mouth is too great to have this be a risk. Take care of your body and know when you're putting toxins on you. The best way to know if they local provider that you're working with is legit, ask them for a tour or just ask for the proof that they're practicing safe business skills.

Finally, understand that it is easy for you to poison yourself if you're not careful in regulating essential oils, These are highly concentrated, potent materials that are diluted for your safety and protection. By taking too much of a pure essence, you could cause serious harm to your body. If something is not working, the solution should never be to keep taking more and upping the dosage without contacting someone who is qualified to council you on the topic first.

Be smart, use your brain and keep it safe. You're using essential oils to be healthy, not to hurt yourself. Keep that in mind.

The Healthy, Natural Way: A Conclusion

So let's sum up everything that we've learned here about essential oils and why you should no longer think of them as snake oil and the people selling them as charlatans looking to leave you with next to nothing, holding the bag and looking for a hand out. In fact, essential oils have a long and respected history among those who have been practicing the medical arts for centuries.

That's where our summary will begin. We learned that essential oils made their appearance in modern writings all the way back in the Middle Ages thanks to the brilliant and advanced work of the Muslim Kingdoms that rose and fell during the period. Regardless of the turmoil that plagued the world back then, Islamic scientists and thinkers continued to pursue the medical studies that have helped progress humanity to the place that we are now.

Though there are ideas that essential oils go as far back as the Romans, this is the first recorded history of essential oils being used in western history. However, in eastern history, it's a quite different story. Medicinal practices have endured and been recorded for a very long time and aromatherapy is still a thriving practice in the Orient. Though controversial, Eastern Medicine has endured to this day and that can't be by accident.

Next we learned how essential oils are made. You were informed that essential oils are made by the utilization of plants that hold medicinal and remedial qualities. The plants are divided up and only certain parts, whether the root or the rhizome, the quality part of the plant is then used to extract essential oils that will help heal and cure whatever ache and pain that you are currently suffering from. There are three methods to getting essential oils and they are expression, distillation, and using solvents to extract the essential oils. They are then diluted and bottled for safe usage for customers all around the world.

We also learned how essential oils are used by those who purchase them. It's important to practice safety when using essential oils and that means taking care not to harm yourself in the event of being allergic or having a negative reaction. However, there are three ways that you can utilize essential oils in your daily life.

The first is by ingesting essential oils through direct usage with capsules or by adding drops of essential oils to your teas. The next practice that you can use is by rubbing essential oils onto parts of your body that are suffering from aches and pains that plague your daily actions.

Finally, the last way for you to utilize essential oils is by inhaling them through placing drops on pieces of cloth, your pillow, your clothes, or in tissues to inhale a few times to clear your sinuses, head, or lungs. Applying essential oils to your daily life is easy and it isn't hard to implement them in your daily life.

Next, I showed you why essential oils are still around with so few people who actually endorse them in the medical community. There is a limited pursuit of understanding and research has left it with relatively small marketing to the rest of the world. But, the market continues to grow and every year those who decide to actually take up essential oils and start using them in daily life. Every year, you will find more and more people using essential oils.

Finally, we discussed how dangerous essential oils can be if there is mishandling and improper use of highly pure essential oils. There are a lot of people who cause harm to themselves and accidentally poison themselves without knowing what they're doing.

It's important to take care of your essential oils and to make sure that insecticides, poisons, or other unnatural compounds are used on some of the source materials. Make sure there at whoever you buy your essential oils from are using regulated, monitored, and completely organic. It's important to keep yourself safe.

So there is all the information that you're going to need to truly introduce yourself to essential oils and make them a part of your life. It's time to start getting ready and using natural solutions to cure your aches and pains, rather than depending upon pharmaceutical companies and their snake oil to help you. Be safe, be smart, and start taking your life into your own hands.

Chapter 21: Rosemary Essential Oil

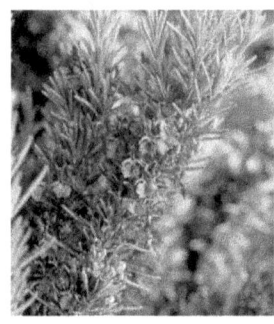

Properties: Rosemary oil is ideal for stirring re-growth, and since a new disinfectant, carminative, antibacterial, as well as analgesic material.

Health benefits: It is rather useful in term of tresses health care, skincare, mouth area health care, anxiousness, mind problem, depressive disorder, ache, frustration, rheumatism, the respiratory system problem, bronchial asthma, indigestion, as well as unwanted wind.

Rosewood essential oil

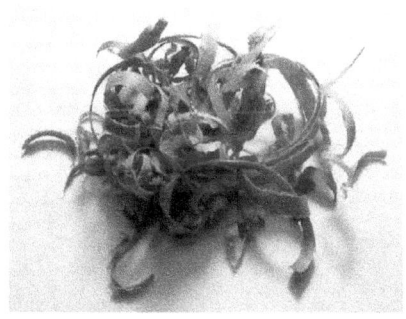

Properties: Rosewood oil is commonly thought of as an analgesic, antiseptic, antibacterial, cephalic, deodorant, insecticide, in addition to stimulant chemical.

Health benefits: It is sometime utilized to lower soreness, combat depression symptom, guard injuries from turning into septic, and boost sexual interest in addition to showcase sex arousal. Additionally, it wipes out bacteria's, in addition to will work for mental performance, whilst recovering headache, traveling away human body odor, eradicating insect pests in addition to stirring gland discharge.

Rue essential oil

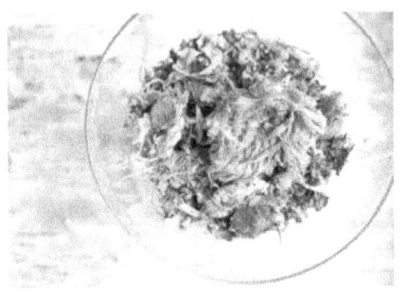

Properties: Bum out over essential oil can be employed as a possible an arthritic, ant rheumatic, antibacterial, insecticidal, plus a dissuasive of numerous worried afflictions.

Health benefits: It can be commonly used to help reduce the effect of the issue associated with toxin, improve the actual flow and also eradication associated with the crystal, stop bacterial and also fungal bacterial infection, wipe out bug, retain nervous feeling steady and also soothes nervous condition. Moreover, the item advance food digestion, eliminate epileptic and also hysteric problem and can possibly help remedy these individual.

Sunflower oil

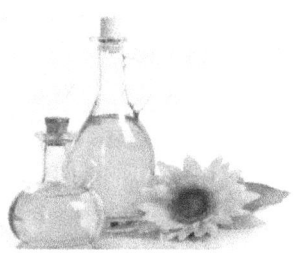

Sunflower oil will be the non-volatile gas condensed by sunflower seed. Sunflower oil is often utilized in food being frying oil, as well as in aesthetic formulations being an emollient. Sunflower oil was first industrially produced in 1835 inside Euro Empire.

Benefits of sunflower oil

Skin Benefits of Sunflower Oil:

Due to its emollient properties, sunflower oil allows your skin layer maintain its wetness. Utilizing sunflower oil as product on the skin color connected with pre-term infants' operates to be a shielding barrier and rubbing all of them with this particular oil allows within lowering skin color illness by means of just about 15 percent. That's why; sunflower oil can be employed inside their day-to-day cosmetic.

Sunflower oil is quite an excellent source of Vitamin E antioxidant with regards to different cosmetic items similar to almond fat as well as Shea butter. Vitamin e antioxidant is essential with regard to protecting against destruction of skin tissues simply by ultraviolet light as well as UVA through the sun. Vitamin E antioxidant increases the design along with health and fitness of one's skin by means of reduction regarding scars along with smoothing regarding recent creases.

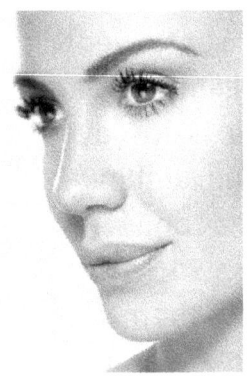

Sunflower oil is also rich in vitamins A, C and D and healthy arytenoids and waxes which form a protective barrier on the skin. So, this particular essential oil is effective in dealing with pimples. Being extremely mild and also non-greasy, it receives assimilated in to the skin tone quickly devoid of clogging or obstructing the particular skin pores. Its array of nutritional vitamins and also essential fatty acids become antioxidants for you to regenerate skin tone tissues and also support your skin layer do away with pimples creating microorganisms.

Beta-carotene can be a thoroughly pigmented fat-soluble chemical substance which can be became Vitamin and mineral any and its particular antioxidant components are usually very therapeutic for the looks of your health and skin. Sunflower acrylic is rich in beta-carotene. Consumption of this kind of chemical substance creates your skin a lesser amount of hypersensitive to the sun. The particular antioxidants in it reduce the effects of the actual no cost radicals that penetrate your skin, producing sunburn along with varieties of sun injury for example skin cancer.

The antioxidant qualities of sunflower essential oil assist in preventing premature indication of ageing. Experience of free radical and sunshine boost the price of ageing of skin color, triggering the event of creases and good lines young. The antioxidant inside sunflower essential oil cheaper danger of developing premature indications of ageing.

Staying by natural mean emollient, sunflower oil help the skin's dampness maintenance capability and is also necessary for those that have dried, dried up as well as hyper-sensitive pore and skin. A combination of sunflower and also castor gas works well making your skin flexible and also taking away expended tissue and also impurities. That blend can be employed to be a solution and also you don't have to utilize a moisturizer because the oils contain fatty acid and also vitamin products to help moisturize your skin.

Sunflower seed essential oil can be an essential oil associated with high-quality since it is usually lighting with surface and very suited to eyes as well as natural skin care. It can be suited to normal to help dried up skin and it is progressively used in aromatherapy because of its gentle aroma as well as lighting surface. It can be used in skin items as well as generates a new gentle feel for the skin.

Hair Benefits of Sunflower Oil:

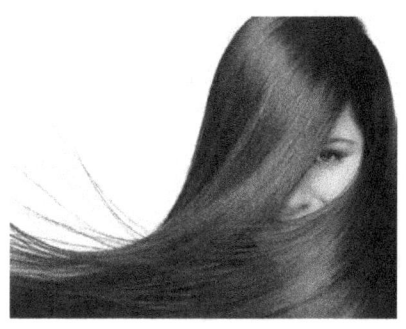

Due to its gentle structure and also slight flavor, sunflower oil softens the actual head of hair and also adds an enjoyable sheen into it. Sunflower seed oil allows you handle frizz, tackle dryness and also destruction and also force you to head of hair workable. That flexible oil preserve your current hair's hold on their owner and also structure and also can be employed like a healthy conditioner. Sunflower oil might be applied and also massaged on the scalp previous to a shower once every seven day pertaining to greatest reward.

Staying very light-weight, sunflower essential oil helps inside treatment muck tresses. The idea nourishes the particular tresses along with stop the break point.

Sunflower oil is an essential cause of gamma leader linolenic acidity (GLA) which often helps within stopping thinning associated with hair. It is efficient within dealing with hair-loss, baldness in addition to alopecia aerate, seen as a spherical patches associated with lost hair.

Other benefits of sunflower oil:

Sunflower gas is made up of selenium that's effective in reducing the chance involving cardiac issue in addition to hepatic destruction. Advanced involving selenium with your our blood can be critical in reducing the chance involving lung in addition to skin varieties of cancer.

The Vitamin supplements M articles involving sunflower fat promotes proper anxious technique, proper digestive system as well as is an excellent cause of energy.

Sunflower oil in addition include healthy protein that happen to be crucial with regard to developing in addition to mending cells in addition to production connected with bodily hormone in addition to digestive enzymes. Our own body requires excessive amount of healthy protein. Since physique isn't going to keep healthy protein, the item need to be taken, in addition to sunflower oil satisfies this kind of prerequisite. Sunflower oil also is made up of zinc which often allow within keeping a normal body's defense mechanism as well as within the curing regarding pain. A different benefit for zinc will be which it keep your feeling regarding stench as well as taste.

Sage essential oil

Properties: Sage oil is generally thought to be an antifungal, antibacterial, antiseptic, antioxidant, cholagogue and choler tic. It's also widely used as a cicatrizing, depurative, digestive system, emenagogue, expectorant, laxative, and a stimulant chemical.

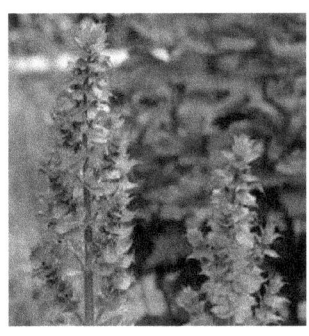

Health benefits: It is seen to lessen virus-like, microbial, fungal along with parasitic microbe infection, and therefore guard's wound against growing to be septic, rehab problem carried out by simply oxidation, soothes swelling, clear spasm, improve the generation connected with bile, along with stimulate digestive function. Moreover, it tiff microbe infection, open upward blocked menstruation, solution cough along with cold, decrease a fever, help clear this bowel, encourage discharge along with commonly improve systemic characteristics.

Sandalwood essential oil

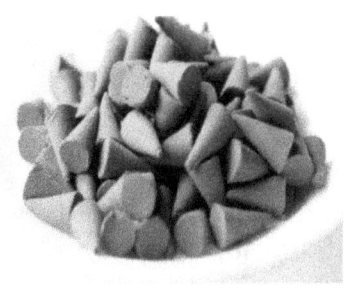

Properties: It might be utilized as an antiseptic, anti-inflammatory, antichloristic, antispasmodic, astringent, carminative, diuretic, disinfectant, emollient, expectorant, hypertensive, memory space increaser, sedative along with a tonic compound.

Health benefits: Sandalwood gas protect injuries via contamination, soothes inflammation on account of nausea and other condition, clear way up muscle spasm, tighten gums and muscle tissue and assist cease hair loss.

It can also slow up the probability of hemorrhaging, recover surgical mark and following represent, provide rest from petrol, increase urination, battle transmission, also it continue epidermis easy & free of transmission. Last but not least, sandalwood gas ordinarily a solution cough and a cold, decrease bloodstream pressure, boost storage, soothes nervous issue and inflammation, and enhance your defense mechanism.

Spearmint essential oil

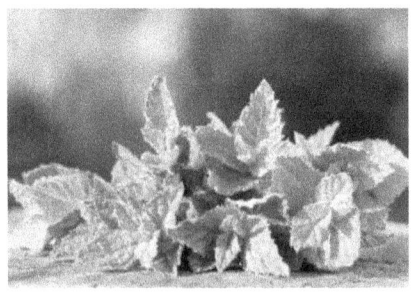

Properties: Spearmint gas is definitely an antiseptic, antispasmodic, carminative, cephalic, emenagogue, insecticide, restorative healing, and also stirring chemical.

Health benefits: It has been used to safeguard pain coming from growing to be septic, clear fits, offer rest from fuel, is useful for serotonin level, start way up blocked menses, get rid of pesky insect, restore health and repair general deterioration, although rousing discharge as well as systemic capabilities.

Spikenard essential oil

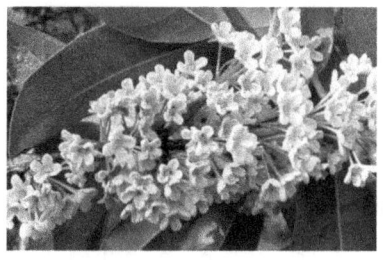

Properties: Spikenard can be deodorant, sedative and also a uterine material.

Health benefits: Traditionally, additionally, it suppresses microbial in addition to yeast increase, sedate inflammation, reduce human body scent, clear bowel, and soothes irritation in addition to tense ailment, whilst repairing uterine well being.

Tagetes essential oil

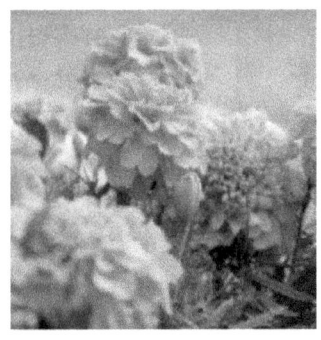

Properties: Tagetes essential oil is definitely an antibiotic, antimicrobial, antiseptic, antispasmodic, disinfectant, insecticide and also a sedative material.

Health benefits: It's popular for you to inhibit biotic, microbial and also other parasitic increase, protect against sepsis, unwind fits, struggle bacterial infection, even though additionally eradicating & repelling insect pest, comforting redness and also anxious ailment.

Tangerine essential oil

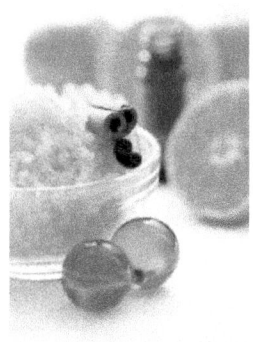

Properties: This kind of essential oil is an antiseptic, antispasmodic, and depurative, sedative, stomachic as well as tonic kind of material.

Health benefits: It really is very popular to shield toward sepsis, encourage increase along with regeneration regarding solar cell, whilst also cleansing the particular our blood, comforting inflammation along with lowering tense disease.

Tansy essential oil

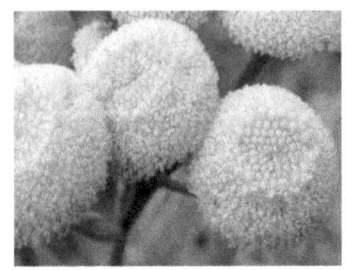

Properties: Tansy fat is an antibacterial, antifungal, anti-inflammatory, antihistaminic, antiviral, febrifuge, insecticide, hormone stimulant, sedative and also a vermifuge substance.

Health benefits: It can be typically accustomed to slow down microbe, fungal along with viral increase, sedate inflammation, curb creation involving histamine and it offer respite from allergic symptom. It is accustomed to lessen fever, destroy & repel pesky insect, encourage the particular creation involving bodily hormone, temporarily relieve inflammation along with resolve nervous hardship.

Tarragon essential oil

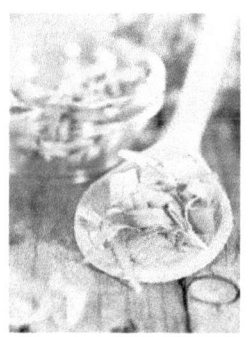

Properties: Tarragon fat is surely an aperitif, circulatory real estate agent, digestive, deodorant, emenagogue, stimulant and also a vermifuge.

Health benefits: This fat in addition treat rheumatism along with joint disease, increase appetite, enhance blood flow along with lymph, help digestion, reduce physique stench, reduce impeded menstruation along with adjust the actual period, induce systemic feature along with wipe out intestinal red worm.

Thuja essential oil

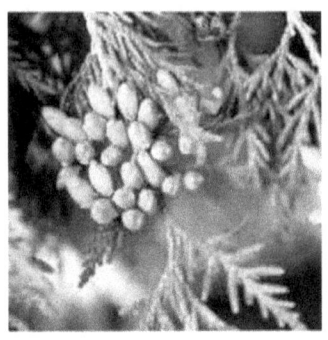

Properties: This sort of gas is definitely an astringent, diuretic, emenagogue, expectorant, pest resistant, stimulant, tonic as well as a vermifuge compound.

Health benefits: It is often very popular to manage rheumatism as well as rheumatoid arthritis, tighten up gum as well as muscle tissue, and also and help to quit hair loss. This minimize the prospect of hemorrhage, will increase urination as well as treatment of toxic compound, minimizes impeded menstruation as well as handle your period, expel phlegm & catarrh, repel insect pest, bring shade toward skin, influence systemic characteristics, as well as usually tone up the entire body.

Thyme essential oil

Properties: This sort of oil is an antispasmodic, ant rheumatic, germ-free, bactericidal, be chic, heart, carminative, diuretic, emenagogue, expectorant, hypertensive, insect poison, stimulant, tonic, and substance.

Health benefits: It can be utilized to dispense with fits, give alleviation from ailment by uprooting poison, secure wound from getting to be septic, and it eliminate microscopic organism. Thyme key oil serve to cure midsection contamination, hack and cold, is useful for heart wellbeing, give alleviation from overabundance gas, mend scar and after imprint, expand pee, control menstrual cycle, and cure hack and cold.

Tuberose essential oil

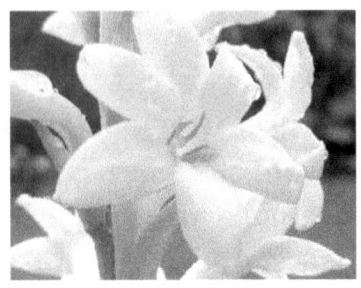

Properties: Tuberose vital oil is ordinarily utilized as a Spanish fly, antiperspirant, unwinding, narcotic and a warming substance.

Health benefits: The oil can improve the charisma, dispense with body smell, unwind the body and psyche, relieve irritation, and lessen anxious issue.

Vanilla essential oil

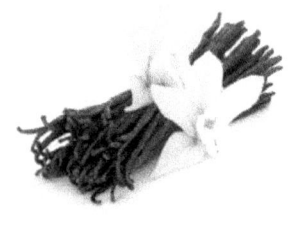

Conclusion

With everything you have hopefully learned from this guide, the next step is to put the above information to practical use, and to try and build your knowledge of essential oils even further. Be sure to keep an eye out for our more detailed guides on aromatherapy and other natural health remedies, targeted at more experienced users.

Take a few months now to build your collection of oils, gain some experience and begin to understand how the individual oils effect you. Once you feel confident with the common essential oils, begin to branch out and utilize the less common but equally effective essential oils out there.

While essential oils are generally thought of as a safer option to potentially harmful and toxic prescriptions, safety is still an issue. These powerful oils are actually concentrated, which can lead to serious damage to your health if not used properly and responsibly. To show you just how concentrated these oils are; it takes a whopping 256 pounds of peppermint leaves to get a mere 1 pound of its essential oil. Now that is some powerfully concentrated oil! Because of the high level of concentration, you really only need to use a small amount of the oil. Furthermore, almost all essential oils should be diluted if it will come in contact with the skin.

Some essential oils — such as orange, lemon, lime, grapefruit and bergamot — cause the skin to become more sensitive to sunlight (UV light). This condition is known as photosensitivity and can cause blistering and discoloration to the skin. It can also leave your skin more susceptible to burning from the sun. In order to avoid photosensitivity, never apply essential oils known to cause this problem within a 12 hour period when your skin will become exposed to sunlight.

Most experts would suggest that you avoid using essential oils on babies and children unless you get the okay from a trusted doctor. If you do use essential oils on your little ones, always exercise extreme caution and dilute the oils more so than you would for an adult. The skin of babies and children are more sensitive than that of an adult, and essential oils that are safe can actually damage their skin. However, there are a few essential oils that experts agree are safe, if used properly, for use on babies and children. These oils include chamomile, lavender, frankincense, lemon and orange. With that said, you should never use peppermint, eucalyptus, wintergreen or rosemary essential oil on babies and children.

Essential oils should be avoided when pregnant or nursing. This is because essential oils have shown to have an effect on hormones, gut bacteria and various other important body aspects that may be harmful or dangerous to the baby in the womb. If, however, you decide to go ahead and use essential oils during this time, you must always proceed with extreme caution. And never use any essential oils without first getting the okay from your doctor.

With that said, there are several oils that experts agree are not safe for use at any time during pregnancy, and should never be used. Rosemary, sage, cinnamon, basil, angelica, black pepper, aniseed, Clary sage, chamomile, camphor, clove, fennel, ginger, horseradish, mustard, jasmine, juniper, nutmeg, mug wart, peppermint, marjoram, myrrh, thyme and wintergreen are among the essential oils that pregnant women should avoid at all

A good general rule of thumb is to talk to your doctor or midwife about essential oils before using if pregnant or nursing. They will be able to give you their expert opinion on whether or not an essential oil should be used.

Keep in mind that not every brand of essential oil is created equal and you should always aim to use high quality oils from a reputable merchant. Furthermore, you should only use therapeutic grade or organic 100- percent pure essential oils. These oils are created using non-chemical process — such as steam distillation — and are considered safe to use both internally and externally.

www.ingramcontent.com/pod-product-compliance
Lightning Source LLC
LaVergne TN
LVHW011936070526
838202LV00054B/4678